国家卫生健康委员会"十三五"规划教材

全国高等中医药教育教材

供中医学、针灸推拿学、中西医临床医学等专业用

中 医 英 语

主　审　方廷钰

主　编　吴　青　龚长华

副主编　肖　平　李涛安　陈　骥　周　恩　何占义

编　者（按姓氏笔画排序）

王科军（滨州医学院）　　　　何占义（长春中医药大学）

叶　晓（浙江中医药大学）　　汶　希（西安工业大学）

田开宇（河南中医药大学）　　陈　战（山东中医药大学）

李晓莉（北京中医药大学）　　陈　骥（成都中医药大学）

李涛安（江西中医药大学）　　周　恩（上海中医药大学）

杨　毅（天津中医药大学）　　徐立群（南京中医药大学）

肖　平（湖南中医药大学）　　龚长华（广东药科大学）

吴　青（北京中医药大学）

人民卫生出版社

·北京·

图书在版编目（CIP）数据

中医英语 / 吴青，龚长华主编 . —北京：人民卫
生出版社，2023.5（2025.2 重印）
ISBN 978-7-117-22598-4

Ⅰ. ①中… Ⅱ. ①吴… ②龚… Ⅲ. ①中国医药学 –
英语 – 中医学院 – 教材 Ⅳ. ①R2

中国国家版本馆 CIP 数据核字（2023）第 036766 号

人卫智网	www.ipmph.com	医学教育、学术、考试、健康， 购书智慧智能综合服务平台
人卫官网	www.pmph.com	人卫官方资讯发布平台

中 医 英 语
Zhongyi Yingyu

主 　编：吴 　青 　龚长华
出版发行：人民卫生出版社（中继线 010-59780011）
地 　　址：北京市朝阳区潘家园南里 19 号
邮 　　编：100021
E - mail：pmph @ pmph.com
购书热线：010-59787592 　010-59787584 　010-65264830
印 　　刷：三河市宏达印刷有限公司
经 　　销：新华书店
开 　　本：787×1092 　1/16 　印张：17
字 　　数：392 千字
版 　　次：2023 年 5 月第 1 版
印 　　次：2025 年 2 月第 2 次印刷
标准书号：ISBN 978-7-117-22598-4
定 　　价：59.00 元
打击盗版举报电话：010-59787491 　E-mail：WQ @ pmph.com
质量问题联系电话：010-59787234 　E-mail：zhiliang @ pmph.com
数字融合服务电话：4001118166 　E-mail：zengzhi @ pmph.com

修订说明

为了更好地贯彻落实《国家中长期教育改革和发展规划纲要(2010—2020)》《医药卫生中长期人才发展规划(2011—2020)》《中医药发展战略规划纲要(2016—2030年)》和《国务院办公厅关于深化高等学校创新创业教育改革的实施意见》精神,做好新一轮全国高等中医药教育教材建设工作,全国高等医药教材建设研究会、人民卫生出版社在教育部、国家卫生和计划生育委员会、国家中医药管理局的领导下,在上一轮教材建设的基础上,组织和规划了全国高等中医药教育本科国家卫生和计划生育委员会"十三五"规划教材的编写和修订工作。

本轮教材修订之时,正值我国高等中医药教育制度迎来60周年之际,为做好新一轮教材的出版工作,全国高等医药教材建设研究会、人民卫生出版社在教育部高等中医学本科教学指导委员会和第二届全国高等中医药教育教材建设指导委员会的大力支持下,先后成立了第三届全国高等中医药教育教材建设指导委员会、首届全国高等中医药教育数字教材建设指导委员会和相应的教材评审委员会,以指导和组织教材的遴选、评审和修订工作,确保教材编写质量。

根据"十三五"期间高等中医药教育教学改革和高等中医药人才培养目标,在上述工作的基础上,全国高等医药教材建设研究会和人民卫生出版社规划、确定了首批中医学(含骨伤方向)、针灸推拿学、中药学、护理学4个专业(方向)89种国家卫生和计划生育委员会"十三五"规划教材。教材主编、副主编和编委的遴选按照公开、公平、公正的原则,在全国50所高等院校2400余位专家和学者申报的基础上,2200位申报者经教材建设指导委员会、教材评审委员会审定和全国高等医药教材建设研究会批准,聘任为主审、主编、副主编、编委。

本套教材主要特色包括以下九个方面:

1. **定位准确,面向实际** 教材的深度和广度符合各专业教学大纲的要求和特定学制、特定对象、特定层次的培养目标,紧扣教学活动和知识结构,以解决目前各院校教材使用中的突出问题为出发点和落脚点,对人才培养体系、课程体系、教材体系进行充分调研和论证,使之更加符合教改实际、适应中医药人才培养要求和市场需求。

2. **夯实基础,整体优化** 以培养高素质、复合型、创新型中医药人才为宗旨,以体现中医药基本理论、基本知识、基本思维、基本技能为指导,对课程体系进行充分调研和认真分析,以科学严谨的治学态度,对教材体系进行科学设计、整体优化,教材编写综合考虑学科的分化、交叉,既要充分体现不同学科自身特点,又应当注意各学科之间有机衔接;确保理论体系完善,知识点结合完备,内容精练、完整,概念准确,切合教学实际。

3. **注重衔接,详略得当** 严格界定本科教材与职业教育教材、研究生教材、毕业后教育教材的知识范畴,认真总结、详细讨论现阶段中医药本科各课程的知识和理论框架,使其在教材中得以凸显,既要相互联系,又要在编写思路、框架设计、内容取舍等方面有一定的区分度。

4. 注重传承,突出特色 本套教材是培养复合型、创新型中医药人才的重要工具,是中医药文明传承的重要载体,传统的中医药文化是国家软实力的重要体现。因此,教材既要反映原汁原味的中医药知识,培养学生的中医思维,又要使学生中西医学融会贯通,既要传承经典,又要创新发挥,体现本版教材"重传承、厚基础、强人文、宽应用"的特点。

5. 纸质数字,融合发展 教材编写充分体现与时代融合、与现代科技融合、与现代医学融合的特色和理念,适度增加新进展、新技术、新方法,充分培养学生的探索精神、创新精神;同时,将移动互联、网络增值、慕课、翻转课堂等新的教学理念和教学技术、学习方式融入教材建设之中,开发多媒体教材、数字教材等新媒体形式教材。

6. 创新形式,提高效用 教材仍将传承上版模块化编写的设计思路,同时图文并茂、版式精美;内容方面注重提高效用,将大量应用问题导入、案例教学、探究教学等教材编写理念,以提高学生的学习兴趣和学习效果。

7. 突出实用,注重技能 增设技能教材、实验实训内容及相关栏目,适当增加实践教学学时数,增强学生综合运用所学知识的能力和动手能力,体现医学生早临床、多临床、反复临床的特点,使教师好教、学生好学、临床好用。

8. 立足精品,树立标准 始终坚持中国特色的教材建设的机制和模式;编委会精心编写,出版社精心审校,全程全员坚持质量控制体系,把打造精品教材作为崇高的历史使命,严把各个环节质量关,力保教材的精品属性,通过教材建设推动和深化高等中医药教育教学改革,力争打造国内外高等中医药教育标准化教材。

9. 三点兼顾,有机结合 以基本知识点作为主体内容,适度增加新进展、新技术、新方法,并与劳动部门颁发的职业资格证书或技能鉴定标准和国家医师资格考试有效衔接,使知识点、创新点、执业点三点结合;紧密联系临床和科研实际情况,避免理论与实践脱节、教学与临床脱节。

本轮教材的修订编写,教育部、国家卫生和计划生育委员会、国家中医药管理局有关领导和教育部全国高等学校本科中医学教学指导委员会、中药学教学指导委员会等相关专家给予了大力支持和指导,得到了全国50所院校和部分医院、科研机构领导、专家和教师的积极支持和参与,在此,对有关单位和个人表示衷心的感谢!希望各院校在教学使用中以及在探索课程体系、课程标准和教材建设与改革的进程中,及时提出宝贵意见或建议,以便不断修订和完善,为下一轮教材的修订工作奠定坚实的基础。

全国高等医药教材建设研究会

人民卫生出版社有限公司

2016 年 3 月

前　言

　　教育部《大学英语教学指南》指出:大学英语教学的主要内容可分为通用英语、专门用途英语和跨文化交际三个部分,由此形成相应的三大类课程。《中医英语》属于专门用途英语教材,在锻炼学生通用英语语言能力基础上,培养学生专业英语运用能力。

　　本教材融中医基本内容与当下中医热点问题于一体,涵盖中医概论、中医核心理念、中医诊断与治则、针灸与推拿、中医预防与治疗、中医养生、中医海外发展以及中医从业人员伦理道德素养等话题,介绍中医相关内容,具有一定的系统性和时代特色,能够较好地满足全国各高等中医院校不同专业背景学生的需要。

　　本教材每个单元内容均围绕主题(theme)设置,突出中医专业英语特点,帮助学生掌握必要的中医(或医学)英语词汇,从词/短语—短句—段落/篇章逐渐递进学习,培养学生中医英语听、说、读、写、译等语言技能,练习设计兼顾中医英语水平测试要求,着重培养学生围绕中医基本内容进行沟通的交流能力,帮助学生奠定学术英语基础,以便顺利进入更高层次的专业英语学习。

　　本教材包括 8 个单元,每个单元均主要涵盖四个模块:听说模块、阅读模块、写译模块和反思模块。

　　1. 听说模块　此模块是课文学习的热身练习,旨在培养学生的中医英语听说能力。此模块由三部分组成:①Before you listen:提供了听力材料中出现的生词;②While you listen:设计了 10 个听力填空;③After you listen:提供了与单元主题内容有关的 2 个讨论题。

　　听说模块旨在为学生创造一个"以听促说,听说结合"的锻炼机会,授课教师可以根据本校具体情况(如课时安排、资源条件、学生的语言基础等)灵活处理这部分教学内容。

　　2. 阅读模块　阅读模块包含 Text A 和 Text B 两篇文章,每篇文章的篇幅在 1000 个英文单词左右,旨在为学生提供地道的语言输入,帮助学生熟悉中医(或医学)专业词汇以及一些基本概念和观点的英语表达。

　　(1) Text A 可作为精读,教师可重点讲授;Text B 可由学生自主学习,教师督促检查。教材在 Text A 和 Text B 课文之后均提供了常用医学词汇前缀、后缀、词根及其意义的说明,并设有巩固练习。

　　(2) Text A 的练习中特别设计了小组讨论练习和模仿句子翻译练习,前者旨在培养学生具备分析、联系、阐释和评价等可迁移性技能(transferable skills),后者旨在帮助学生在课文主题及句型基础上能够准确地完成中译英练习,提高语言输出能力。

　　3. 写译模块　结合单元主题,设置相应写译专题,锻炼学生英语遣词造句和写译技能。内容包括:①介绍中医;②中医术语定义;③描述中医证候;④描述艾灸使用方法;⑤提供中医建议;⑥介绍中医养生方法;⑦描述海外中医发展;⑧撰写中医伦理准则。

　　写译模块结合阅读文章,注重实用性,通过"要点讲解"—"输入"(单句)—"输入"(范文）—"输出"（句子翻译）—"输出"（短文写作)5个步骤,培养学生中医英语写作技能与中医话题拓展能力。

4. 反思模块　该模块是单元主题再拓展环节,在整个单元语言输入和语言输出练习之后,为师生提供讨论素材,培养学生中医话题英语思辨能力(critical thinking ability)。内容涉及:①中医国际化背景下语言媒介的作用;②中医名词术语表达标准化;③中医辨证论治的重要性;④针灸的国际传播;⑤中医疾病预防的优势;⑥公众对中医养生的热衷;⑦海外中医立法问题;⑧跨文化医务沟通。

围绕某个既定话题,有两方面教学重点:第一,说什么;第二,怎么说。"说什么"指引导学生掌握谋篇布局或话语结构,清楚列出陈述思路和重点内容。"怎么说"指帮助学生掌握必要的句型结构和术语词汇。通过上述两方面的重点训练,培养学生具有较强的中医英语讲述能力。

由于中医术语翻译尚有许多不确定的方面,本书只对很少一部分的术语进行了统一改写。例如,"中医"的译名采用 traditional Chinese medicine,简称为 TCM(不含引用的原文题目或网址名称;此外,如果原作者使用了 Chinese medicine,编者予以保留,未做改写);"证"的译名采用 pattern;"虚"的译名采用 deficiency,"实"的译名采用 excess;"经络"的译名采用 meridian;古籍《黄帝内经》的译名采用 *Huangdi's Inner Canon of Medicine*。其余术语名称全书未做统一调整,留待读者进一步权衡、思考。

本教材在编写过程中得到了国内各参编院校和国外中医机构和中医专业人士的大力支持。在编写的过程中,我们参考了国内外大量的英文文献资料,在此对这些文献资料的作者及出版机构表示衷心的感谢！来自加拿大的 Suzanne Robidoux(苏璇)博士为本教材的英语听力音频进行了专业录制,在此对她表示衷心的感谢！本书在校稿过程中得到了北京中医药大学人文学院中医药外语专业研究生凌武娟、张晶、周阿剑、张千的帮助。感谢北京中医药大学人文学院都立澜教授、李晓莉副教授、成都中医药大学陈骥教授和天津中医药大学杨毅副教授积极试用本教材。最后,衷心感谢教材主审方廷钰教授,他严谨的治学态度以及对中医英语的热爱令同行后辈敬仰,我们从他的审校批阅中受益匪浅。

本教材适用于全国高等中医院校大学本科二年级及以上学生使用。根据大多数院校大学英语课时的设置习惯和学生英语水平,本教材的教学时数设定为 36~54 学时。

编　者
2022 年 3 月

Contents

Unit 1

An Overview of Traditional Chinese Medicine

LEARNING OUTCOMES

This unit offers you opportunities to:
- **define** traditional Chinese medicine (TCM)
- **outline** the history of TCM
- **explain** the fundamental concepts and framework of TCM
- **understand** the fundamental differences between TCM and Western medicine
- **reflect on** the role of English language in the dissemination of TCM culture

笔记

PART I　LISTENING AND SPEAKING

Before you listen

In this section you will hear a short passage entitled "What Is Traditional Chinese Medicine". The following words and phrases may be of help.

incorporate /ɪnˈkɔːpəreɪt/	vt.	包含；吸收；合并
therapy /ˈθerəpi/	n.	治疗
practitioner /prækˈtɪʃ(ə)nə/	n.	执业医生；从业者（尤指律师、医师）
unobstructed /ˌʌnəbˈstrʌktɪd/	a.	不被阻塞的，畅通无阻的
meridian /məˈrɪdɪən/	n.	（中医学）经，经络
disruption /dɪsˈrʌpʃn/	n.	紊乱，失调
circulation /ˌsəːkjʊˈleɪʃ(ə)n/	n.	血液循环
chronic /ˈkrɒnɪk/	a.	慢性的；长期的
metabolic /ˌmetəˈbɒlɪk/	a.	新陈代谢的
degenerative /dɪˈdʒen(ə)rətɪv/	a.	退步的，变质的，退化的
arthritis /ɑːˈθraɪtɪs/	n.	关节炎
formula /ˈfɔːmjʊlə/	n.	配方，处方；方剂（中医学）
allergy /ˈælədʒi/	n.	变态反应，过敏
asthma /ˈæsmə/	n.	哮喘
reinforce healthy qi to eliminate pathogenic factors		扶正祛邪

While you listen

Listen to the passage carefully and fill in each of the blanks marked from 1) to 10) according to what you have heard.

What Is Traditional Chinese Medicine?

ER-1-1
Listening
practice

　　Traditional Chinese medicine (TCM), incorporating different therapies, has been evolving for more than 2,000 years before it gains its status as an independent healing system. One of its 1)＿＿＿＿＿ is to "reinforce healthy qi to eliminate pathogenic factors". TCM not only treats illness, but also emphasizes the defense function and the recovering and healing 2)＿＿＿＿＿ of the human body. The primary objective of TCM is to 3)＿＿＿＿＿.

　　TCM takes 4)＿＿＿＿＿ functioning of body, mind and spirit as the key to health. TCM doctors and 5)＿＿＿＿＿ hold that health depends on the 6)＿＿＿＿＿ flow

2

of qi along meridians, while disease is the result of 7)＿＿＿＿＿＿ in the circulation of qi.

TCM is especially effective for 8)＿＿＿＿＿＿ and complex diseases including metabolic diseases, degenerative conditions (such as knee arthritis) and age-related diseases. Nowadays, 9)＿＿＿＿＿＿ on the effectiveness of TCM are being 10)＿＿＿＿＿＿ not only in China but also in many other countries. For example, TCM herbal formulas for treating allergy and asthma are under intensive study in the U.S.

After you listen

Please discuss with your partner the following questions and give your presentation to the class.

1) What do you know about TCM as a healing system in terms of its history, guiding principles, effectiveness, etc.?

2) From the perspective of TCM, what is disease and what is health? How is it related to the concept of health proposed by the World Health Organization?

PART II　READING

Text A

An Introduction to Traditional Chinese Medicine

1　Traditional Chinese medicine (TCM) is a system of diagnosis and health care that has evolved over thousands of years. It **encompasses** many different practices, including **acupuncture**, **moxibustion**, Chinese herbal medicine, tuina-massage, **dietary** therapy, qigong, etc.

2　The first documented TCM **monograph**, *Huangdi Neijing* (*Huangdi's Inner Canon of Medicine*)[①] was written approximately between 770 BC and 200 BC. The main achievement of this book is that it establishes the basic theoretical framework of TCM such as *zangxiang xueshuo* (the theory of visceral **manifestations**), *jing qi shen xueshuo* (the theory of essence, qi and spirit), *yinyang wuxing xueshuo* (the theory of yin-yang and the five phases), and *jingluo xueshuo* (the theory of meridians and collaterals).

3　It is important to understand how historical factors have impacted on the establishment of the TCM theory. During the period between 770 BC and 200 BC when *Huangdi's Inner Canon of Medicine* was written, science and technology around the world was still in its **naive** form; therefore, the study of medicine would not be carried out by **sophisticated** experiments, and rather it was via direct observation and clinical practice. The basic TCM theory was generated by the involvement of ancient Chinese philosophies such as the Daoist school[②] and **Confucianism** (to name a few but not limited to this), to **induct** and **deduct** the section of the knowledge and experiences that came from the observation and clinical practices. These TCM theories have been used as guidelines for clinical practice and at the same time were tested so that, eventually, by dumping incorrect and **incoherent** knowledge or theory, they were **converted** into a better form of TCM theory. There are obviously marked connections that can be identified between ancient Chinese philosophies and TCM theory, for example, from the harmony between man and nature of the Daoist school and Confucianism to the **holistic** approach concept of TCM, and from *zhongyong zhi dao* (the doctrine of the golden **mean**) to the harmony among the *zang-fu* organs, qi-blood and yin-yang.

4　Built upon the TCM theory and knowledge in and before the Han Dynasty (206 BC–220 AD), *Shanghan Zabing Lun* (***Treatise** on Cold-**induced** and **Miscellaneous** Diseases*) was written around 210 AD by Zhang Zhongjing. Later, the book was divided into two

---

① *Huangdi Neijing* (*Huangdi's Inner Canon of Medicine*):《黄帝内经》,又译为 *Huangdi's Internal Classic*,是我国现存最早的中医典籍。

② the Daoist school: 道家学派。

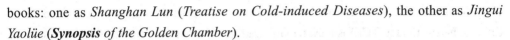

books: one as *Shanghan Lun* (*Treatise on Cold-induced Diseases*), the other as *Jingui Yaolüe* (**Synopsis** *of the Golden Chamber*).

5　Being the father of TCM, Zhang Zhongjing made great contributions to TCM in the following aspects: first, the establishment of *bianzheng lunzhi* (**differentiation** of patterns and treatment[①])—the clinical **methodology**; second, the establishment of the Eight **Therapeutic** Methods, which includes **diaphoresis**, **emetic** method, **purgative** therapy, harmonizing, warming method, heat clearing, **tonification**, and resolving therapy. In line with the therapeutic methods, 269 herbal **prescriptions** were recorded in his books. The above clinical methodologies are still considered to be the most valuable ones and are used as the guidelines for clinical work nowadays. Zhang Zhongjing's **herbal** prescriptions are considered to be the classic herbal prescriptions of TCM.

6　In the Qing Dynasty, two TCM masters deserve the most **credit** in developing the theoretical framework of TCM for the **diagnosis** and treatment of **infectious** diseases. One is Ye Tianshi, who wrote *Wenre Lun* (*Treatise on Warm-heat Diseases*) and developed *wei qi ying xue bianzheng*[②] (differentiation of patterns by analysis of the condition of the defensive, qi, nutritive and blood levels). The other is Wu Jutong, who wrote *Wenbing Tiaobian* (*The Differentiation of* **Epidemic Febrile** *Diseases*) and set up *sanjiao bianzheng* (pattern differentiation according to the theory of *sanjiao*). Their clinical methodologies are widely accepted and have become the guidelines for clinical practice dealing with epidemic febrile diseases.

7　After the founding of the People's Republic of China in 1949, the central government gave its **priority** to the expansion of TCM. The first four TCM colleges were established in 1956, with every province later getting their own TCM colleges. The establishment of TCM colleges indicates that the TCM education model has changed from traditional **apprenticeship**-style teaching to the modern standard education model. This not only enables graduates from TCM colleges to have knowledge in both TCM and **biomedicine** and later become the **backbone** of TCM hospitals, but also enables scientific researches to be carried out on TCM.

8　Some well-developed **affiliated** hospitals of TCM colleges/universities not only have been equipped with the **state-of-the-art** equipment, but also with the **expertise** in both TCM and biomedicine.

9　As one of the TCM **modalities**, acupuncture was introduced to Western countries in the 1970s. On the one hand, it is pleased to know that the practice of acupuncture has gained popularity since; but on the other hand, it can be **problematic** by only accepting the practical part of acupuncture without bothering to know the theoretical part of TCM. This not only limits acupuncture to achieve its potential clinical outcome, but also **conveys** the wrong information about what TCM is.

---

①　differentiation of patterns and treatment: 辨证论治。"证"有时翻译成 syndrome，其指西医的综合征，建议用 pattern 表达中医的"证"，以示概念上的区别。

②　*Wei Qi Ying Xue Bian Zheng*: 卫气营血辨证。

10　Nowadays, TCM is known by Western countries as only acupuncture and some Chinese herbs. In fact, TCM is a systematic traditional **macro** medicine with richness in its contents. Therefore, it is **imperative** to give an appropriate definition in order to gain more understanding of this medicine.

11　TCM is a systematic traditional macro medicine, which uses the TCM theoretical framework to study the living phenomena of human beings, the functions of organs and parts of the body and their interrelationships, and how these functions and interrelationships are affected by **pathogenic** factors. Guided by the theories, TCM treats a variety of diseases by using the Eight Therapeutic Methods with the treatment based on the differentiation of patterns.

Reference: HE J, HOU X Y. The potential contributions of traditional Chinese medicine to emergency medicine. [J/OL]. World journal of emergency medicine, 2013, 4 (2): 92-97, accessed on October 11, 2022 from https://www.ncbi.nlm.nih.gov/pmc/articles/PMC4129829/. DOI: 10.5847/wjem.j.issn.1920-8642.2013.02.002

New words

encompass /ɪnˈkʌmpəs/	*vt.*	include comprehensively 包含, 包括
acupuncture /ˈækjʊˌpʌn(k)tʃə/	*n.*	a system of complementary medicine in which fine needles are inserted in the skin at specific points along what are considered to be lines of energy (meridians), used in the treatment of various physical and mental conditions 针刺
moxibustion /ˌmɒksɪˈbʌstʃ(ə)n/	*n.*	the burning of moxa on or near a person's skin as a counterirritant 艾灸
dietary /ˈdaɪət(ə)ri/	*a.*	relating to or provided by diet 饮食的, 规定食物的
monograph /ˈmɒnəgrɑːf/	*n.*	a detailed written study of a single specialized subject or an aspect of it 专著, 专论
manifestation /ˌmænɪfeˈsteɪʃ(ə)n/	*n.*	a symptom of an ailment 表现, 表现形式
naive /nɑːˈiːv/	*a.*	(of a person) natural and unaffected 天真的, 单纯的
sophisticated /səˈfɪstɪkeɪtɪd/	*a.*	(of a machine, system, or technique) developed to a high degree of complexity (机器、装置等) 高级的, 精密的;(方法) 复杂的
Confucianism /kənˈfjuːʃənɪz(ə)m/	*n.*	a system of philosophical and ethical teachings founded by Confucius and developed by Mencius 儒教, 儒家学说

induct /ɪnˈdʌkt/	vt.	use known facts to produce rules or principles 归纳
deduct /dɪˈdʌkt/	vt.	use the knowledge or information you have to understand something or form an opinion 演绎
incoherent /ˌɪnkə(ʊ)ˈhɪər(ə)nt/	a.	not logical or internally consistent 前后矛盾的,不一致的
convert /kənˈvɜːt/	vt.	change the form, character, or function of sth. 使转变
holistic /həʊˈlɪstɪk/	a.	characterized by the treatment of the whole person, taking into account mental and social factors, rather than just the symptoms of a disease 整体的
mean /miːn/	n.	a condition, quality, or course of action equally removed from two opposite extremes 中间值,平均值
treatise /ˈtriːtɪs/	n.	a written work dealing formally and systematically with a subject 论述;专著
induce /ɪnˈdjuːs/	vt.	bring about or give rise to 引起;导致
miscellaneous /ˌmɪsəˈleɪnɪəs/	a.	(of items or people gathered or considered together) of various types or from different sources 各种各样的;混杂的
synopsis /sɪˈnɒpsɪs/	n.	a brief summary or general survey of sth. 提要,概要
differentiation /ˌdɪfərenʃɪˈeɪʃn/	n.	the action or process of differentiating 辨别
methodology /ˌmeθəˈdɒlədʒi/	n.	a system of methods used in a particular area of study or activity (从事某一活动的)一套方法;方法论;方法学
therapeutic /ˌθerəˈpjuːtɪk/	a.	relating to the healing of disease 治疗(学)的,疗法的
diaphoresis /ˌdaɪəfəˈriːsɪs/	n.	sweating, especially to an unusual degree as a symptom of disease or a side effect of a drug 发汗
emetic /ɪˈmetɪk/	a.	(of a substance) causing vomiting 催吐的
purgative /ˈpɜːɡətɪv/	a.	strongly laxative in effect 通便的,泻下的
	n.	a laxative 泻药(药力强)

tonification /ˌtəʊnɪfɪˈkeɪʃ(ə)n/   *n.*   (of acupuncture or herbal medicine) the effect or the function of increasing the available energy of (a bodily part or system) 补益,强壮

prescription /prɪˈskrɪpʃ(ə)n/   *n.*   an instruction written by a medical practitioner that authorizes a patient to be issued with a medicine or treatment 药方,处方

herbal /ˈhɜːb(ə)l/   *a.*   relating to or made from herbs, especially those used in cooking and medicine 药草的,草本的

credit /ˈkredɪt/   *n.*   public acknowledgement or praise, given or received when a person's responsibility for an action or idea becomes apparent 赞誉

diagnosis /ˌdaɪəgˈnəʊsɪs/   *n.*   the identification of the nature of an illness or other problem by examination of the symptoms 诊断

infectious /ɪnˈfekʃəs/   *a.*   (of a disease or disease-causing organism) liable to be transmitted to people, organism, etc. through the environment 传染的;有传染性的

epidemic /ˌepɪˈdemɪk/   *a.*   (of a disease) with large numbers of cases occurring at the same time in a particular community 流行性的

febrile /ˈfiːbraɪl/   *a.*   having or showing the symptoms of a fever 发热的

priority /praɪˈɒrɪti/   *n.*   the fact or condition of being regarded or treated as more important than others 优先考虑的事;优先,优先权

apprenticeship /əˈprentɪ(s)ʃɪp/   *n.*   employment as an apprentice 学徒工,当学徒;(中医)师承模式

biomedicine /ˌbaɪəʊˈmedsɪn/   *n.*   relating to both biology and medicine 生物医学

backbone /ˈbækbəʊn/   *n.*   the chief support of a system or organization 中坚力量;骨干;支柱

affiliated /əˈfɪlɪeɪtɪd/   *a.*   (of a subsidiary group or a person) officially attached or connected to an organization 隶属的,附属的,有关联的

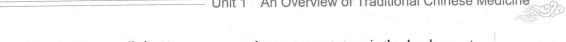

state-of-the-art /ˌsteɪt əv ðɪ ˈɑːt/	a.	the most recent stage in the development of a product, incorporating the newest ideas and features 使用最先进技术的;体现最高水平的
expertise /ˌekspəˈtiːz/	n.	expert skill or knowledge in a particular field 专业知识或技能
modality /mə(ʊ)ˈdælɪti/	n.	a method of therapy that involves physical or electrical therapeutic treatment 治疗方法
problematic /ˌprɒbləˈmætɪk/	a.	constituting or presenting a problem 成问题的,产生问题的
convey /kənˈveɪ/	vt.	make (an idea, impression, or feeling) known or understandable 表达,传达
macro /ˈmækrəʊ/	a.	large-scale; overall 宏观的;全面的
imperative /ɪmˈperətɪv/	a.	of vital importance; crucial 极重要的;必要的
pathogenic /ˌpæθəˈdʒænɪk/	a.	(of a bacterium, virus, or other microorganism) causing disease(细菌、病毒或其他微生物)病原的,致病的

Phrases and expressions

health care	保健
Chinese herbal medicine	中草药,中药
dietary therapy	饮食疗法
five phases	五行
to name a few	举几个例子
but not limited to	但不限于……
induct and deduct	归纳和演绎
clinical practice	临床实践
convert into	转变为,转化为
holistic approach concept	整体观
the doctrine of the golden mean	中庸之道
differentiation of patterns	辨证
in line with	与……一致,符合
therapeutic method	治法
theoretical framework	理论框架
diagnosis and treatment	诊断与治疗
give priority to	认为……优先,优先考虑

笔记

affiliated hospital	附属医院
gain popularity	得到普及
gain (more) understanding of sth.	对……有（更多的）理解，增进理解
pathogenic factor	邪气；致病因素

Task One　Preview

1. Learn the following roots and affixes. Write out the Chinese meaning of the given words.

Roots/Affixes	Meaning of roots/affixes	Words	Chinese meaning of the given words
arthr (o)-	joint	arthritis arthroscopy	_____ _____
bi (o)	life	antibiotic biomedicine	_____ _____
dem (o)	connected with people or population	endemic epidemic	_____ _____
doc-	teach	docile doctrine	_____ _____
en-	put into or on	encompass enroll	_____ _____
exo-	outside, outer	exogenous exoskeleton	_____ _____
-graph	record	radiograph cardiograph	_____ _____
gyn (a)ec (o)-	woman	gynecology gynecopathy	_____ _____
-ics	denoting arts or sciences, branches of study or action	obstetrics pediatrics	_____ _____
meta-	altered	metabolic metagenesis	_____ _____
mill (i)-	thousand	millennium millipede	_____ _____
mono-	one	monologue monomania	_____ _____
- (o)logy	denoting a subject of study or interest	biology pathology	_____ _____

笔记

ot (o)	ear	otology	
		otoscope	
oste (o)	bone	osteoarthritis	
		osteology	
-ous	characterized by; of the nature of	dangerous	
		pathogenous	
path (o)	disease, illness, sickness	pathogen	
		pathologist	
soph	wise	philosophy	
		sophomore	

2. Write down the questions you would like to ask or discuss about the text.

_____

_____

_____

Task Two   Speaking

1. Answer the following questions according to the text.

1) What does TCM generally encompass?

2) What is the significance of *Huangdi's Inner Canon of Medicine* to TCM?

3) What are the connections between ancient Chinese philosophies and TCM theories?

4) Why do people regard Zhang Zhongjing as the father of TCM?

5) Who are the representative figures in developing the theoretical framework of TCM for the diagnosis and treatment of infectious diseases? What are their contributions?

6) What is the significance of establishing TCM colleges in 1956 in China?

7) As one of the TCM modalities, acupuncture was introduced to Western countries in the 1970s. What impact does it have on the development of acupuncture in the West?

8) What is the appropriate definition of TCM to avoid misunderstanding in intercultural communication?

2. Work in pairs or groups and exchange views on the following passage.

Good Medicine Tastes Bitter

Compared to Western medicine, traditional Chinese medicine (TCM) seems a little bit mysterious.

TCM has a systematic tradition of medical science, and theory. There are two renowned classics: *Huangdi's Inner Canon of Medicine* and *Compendium of Materia Medica*. The basic principle of TCM is to prevent disease, and to prioritize maintaining good health; meanwhile, it emphasizes finding a fundamental cure, rather than curing disease superficially. The biggest difference between TCM and Western medicine is that in Western medicine for almost every sickness, doctors prescribe pills for patients, whereas in TCM, effective treatments also include acupuncture, massage, cupping, and *guasha* therapy.

TCM generally regards Western medicine as curing the symptoms but not eliminating the fundamental cause, and also having side effects. However, when they get seriously ill, or need intense treatment, Chinese people may turn to Western medicine or a combination of both Eastern and Western therapies.

The definition of illness is quite different between Chinese and Western doctors. For example, suffering from excessive internal heat in TCM is not the same as fever or inflammation. If a person has excessive internal heat, it means that his body has a yin-yang imbalance. He or she needs to take some herbal medicine, drink tea or change his or her diet to nurse the health and to rid the body from excessive heat and toxic materials.

When someone has a cold or flu, a TCM doctor would advise him or her not to take too much medicine because in TCM theory there is a saying "fighting poison with poison", and sometimes the patient doesn't need medicines but can recover naturally with good rest. Most Chinese don't like to take medicine arbitrarily, because they believe that any medicine is more or less harmful to the body. Therefore, they often remind others to take as little medicine as possible.

Reference: ROUSSILLA S. Good medicine tastes bitter [J]. China today, 2015, (7): 80.

Topic for discussion: Why do Westerners find traditional Chinese medicine a bit mysterious?

Task Three   Vocabulary

1. Match up each word in Column A with its appropriate definition from Column B.

Column A

Column B

1) diaphoresis

a. the effect or the function of increasing the available energy of (a bodily part or system)

2) monograph

b. strongly laxative in effect

3) febrile

c. a written work dealing formally and systematically with a subject

4) meridian

d. a detailed written study of a single specialized subject or an aspect of it

5) holistic

e. having or showing the symptoms of a fever

6) treatise

f. an instruction written by a medical practitioner

7) diagnosis

g. sweating

8) biomedicine

h. each of a set of pathways in the body along which vital energy is said to flow

9) emetic

i. the identification of the nature of an illness or other problem by examination of the symptoms

10) prescription

j. relating to both biology and medicine

11) purgative　　　k. treating the whole person rather than just the symptoms of a disease

12) tonification　　l. causing vomiting

2. Fill in the blanks with the words given below. Change the form where necessary.

as	cast	correspond	ecosystem	force
interact	into	metaphor	microcosm	plant
power	preserve	when	whole	within

Major Concepts of Traditional Chinese Medicine

Traditional Chinese medicine (TCM) rests upon a set of assumptions. Within the Eastern worldview, the human being is a 1)＿＿＿＿＿＿＿, a universe in miniature, the offspring of Heaven and Earth, a fusion of cosmic and terrestrial（地球的）2)＿＿＿＿＿＿＿. People are recognized as beings with a self-aware mind 3)＿＿＿＿＿＿＿ in physical form. The unseen and the seen, psyche（心智,精神）and soma（身体,肉体）, are mutually valid and cogenerative（相生的）.

Whereas Western medicine relies on Cartesian-Newtonian（笛卡尔 - 牛顿理论思想为基础的）science, TCM is embedded 4)＿＿＿＿＿＿＿ a philosophy of nature. A postulate（假设）of TCM is that by observing patterns in the natural world, the dynamics of human nature are known. The world is a single, unbroken 5)＿＿＿＿＿＿＿—Tao—that exists within. Chinese medical logic relies upon correspondence thinking: things that 6)＿＿＿＿＿＿＿ to the same thing correspond to each other. Life arises from the magnetic interplay of the polar forces: yang and yin, Heaven and Earth, heat and cold, sun and shadow, dryness and dampness, summer and winter. Just as these divisions are relational, so all living processes are seen as a mosaic（镶嵌图案）of connected relationships and conditions.

In short, the human body is viewed as a (n) 7)＿＿＿＿＿＿＿, and the language of TCM is based on 8)＿＿＿＿＿＿＿ from nature. Each person has a unique terrain to be mapped, a resilient（能复原的）yet sensitive ecology to be maintained. 9)＿＿＿＿＿＿＿ a gardener adjusts irrigation（灌溉）and applies compost（堆肥）, the traditional Chinese doctor uses acupuncture, herbs, food, etc. to recover and 10)＿＿＿＿＿＿＿ health.

Reference: BEINFIELD H, KORNGOLD E. Chinese traditional medicine: an introductory overview. Altern Ther Health Med, 1995, 1 (1): 44-52.

Task Four　Translation

1. Study the following sentences and pay attention to the underlined parts.

1) The main achievement of this book is that it establishes the basic theoretical framework of TCM. (para. 2)

2) The study of medicine would not be carried out by sophisticated experiments, and rather it was via direct observation and clinical practice. (para. 3)

3) These TCM theories have been used as guidelines for clinical practices. (para. 3)

笔记

4) Being the father of TCM, Zhang Zhongjing made great contributions to TCM <u>in the following aspects</u>. (para. 5)

5) It is pleased to know that the practice of acupuncture has <u>gained popularity</u> since. (para. 9)

6) This not only limits acupuncture to <u>achieve its potential clinical outcome</u>, but also conveys the wrong information about what TCM is. (para. 9)

2. Translate the following sentences into English.

1) 这篇论文为未来的研究建立了理论框架。

2) 中医理论通过直接观察与临床实践逐步形成。

3) 此技术规范是中医医生临床操作的指南。

4) 作为认知心理学（cognitive psychology）之父，奈瑟尔（Neisser）对认知研究做出了如下贡献。

5) 由于疗效显著，中医在世界上越来越受欢迎。

6) 在某种程度上，对中医的误解与限制使其难以获得应有的疗效。

Text B

The Web That Has No Weaver: Understanding Chinese Medicine

1　Chinese medicine is a coherent and independent system of thought and practice that has been developed over two millennia. Based on ancient texts, it is the result of a continuous process of critical thinking, as well as **extensive** clinical observation and testing. It represents a thorough formulation and reformulation of material by respected **clinicians** and theoreticians. It is also, however, rooted in the philosophy, logic, **sensibility**, and habits of a civilization entirely foreign to Westerners. It has therefore developed its own **perception** of health and illness.

2　Chinese medicine considers important certain aspects of the human body and personality that are not significant to Western medicine. At the same time, Western medicine observes and can describe aspects of the human body that are insignificant or not **perceptible** to Chinese medicine. For instance, Chinese medical theory does not have the concept of a nervous system. Nevertheless, evidence exists demonstrating Chinese medicine's capacity to treat some neurological disorders. Similarly, Chinese medicine does not **perceive** an **endocrine** system, yet it treats what Western medicine calls endocrine disorders. Nor does TCM recognize *Streptococcus pneumoniae*[①] as a **pathological** cause

---

① *Streptococcus pneumoniae*: 肺炎链球菌，肺炎双球菌。

14

of **pneumonia**, yet before the discovery of antibiotics, its treatments seemed to offer a reasonable and relatively effective response.

3　Chinese medicine also uses **terminology** that is strange to the Western ear. For example, the Chinese refer to certain diseases as being generated by "dampness", "heat", or "wind". Modern Western medicine does not recognize dampness, yet can treat what Chinese medicine describes as dampness of the spleen. Modern Western medicine does not speak of fire, but can, from a Chinese **perspective**, **stoke** the fire of the kidney or **extinguish** excess fire raging out of control in the lungs. In Western medicine, wind is not considered a disease factor; yet Western medicine is able to prevent liver wind from going to the head, or to extinguish **rampaging** wind in the skin. The perceptions of the two traditions reflect two different worlds, but both can affect and often heal human beings regardless of their cultural affiliation.

4　The difference between the two medicines, however, is greater than that between their descriptive languages. The actual logical structure underlying the methodology, the habitual mental operations that guide the physician's clinical insight and critical judgment, differs radically in the two traditions.

5　The two different logical structures have pointed the two medicines in different directions. Biomedicine, a more accurate name for Western medicine, is primarily concerned with **isolable** disease categories or **agents** of disease, which it zeroes in on, isolates, and tries to change, control, or destroy. An **ontologically circumscribed entity** is the **privileged** ideal of the system. The Western **physician** starts with a symptom, then searches for the underlying mechanism—a **precise** *cause* for a specific *disease*. The disease may affect various parts of the body, but it is relatively a well-defined, **self-contained** phenomenon. Precise diagnosis frames an exact, **quantifiable** description of a narrow area. The physician's logic is analytic—cutting through the **accumulation** of bodily phenomena like a surgeon's **scalpel** to isolate one single entity or cause.

6　The Chinese physician, in contrast, directs his or her attention to the complete **physiological** and psychological individual. All relevant information, including the symptom as well as the patient's other general characteristics, is gathered and woven together until it forms what Chinese medicine calls a "pattern of disharmony". This pattern of disharmony describes a situation of "imbalance" in a patient's body. Oriental diagnostic technique does not turn up a specific disease entity or a precise cause, but **renders** an almost poetic, yet workable, description of a whole person. The question of cause and effect is always secondary to the overall pattern. One does not ask, "What *X* is causing *Y*?" but rather, "What is the relationship between *X* and *Y*?" The Chinese are interested in **discerning** the relationships in human activities occurring at the same time. The logic of Chinese medicine is **organismic** or **synthetic**, attempting to organize symptoms and signs into understandable **configurations**. The total configurations, the patterns of disharmony, provide the framework for treatment. The therapy then attempts to bring the configuration into balance, to restore harmony to the individual.

7　This difference between Western and Eastern perception can be illustrated by portions of clinical studies done in hospitals in China. In a typical study a Western physician, using upper-**gastrointestinal** x-rays or **endoscopy** by means of a **fiberscope**, diagnoses two patients with stomach pain as having **peptic ulcer** disease. From the Western doctor's perspective, based on the analytic tendency to narrow diagnosis to an underlying entity, both patients suffer from the same disorder. The physician then sends the patients to a Chinese doctor for examination. The following results are found.

8　Upon questioning and examining the first patient, the Chinese physician finds pain that increases at touch (by **palpation**) but **diminishes** with the application of cold **compresses**. The patient has a **robust constitution**, broad shoulders, a reddish **complexion**, and a full, deep voice. He seems **assertive** and even **aggressive**. He seems to be challenging the doctor. He is **constipated** and has dark yellow **urine**. His tongue has a greasy yellow coating; his pulse is "full" and "wiry". The Oriental physician characterizes this patient as having the pattern of disharmony called "damp heat affecting the spleen".

9　When the Chinese physician examines the second patient, he finds a different set of signs, which indicate another overall pattern. The patient is thin. Her complexion is **ashen**, though her cheeks are **ruddy**. She is constantly thirsty, her palms are sweaty, and she has a tendency toward constipation and **insomnia**. She seems nervous, **fidgety**, and unable to relax and also complains of feeling pressured. In her life, she is constantly on the go and has been unable to be in a stable relationship. Her tongue is dry and slightly red, with no "**moss**"; her pulse is "thin" and also a bit "fast". This patient is said to have the pattern of "deficient yin affecting the stomach", a disharmony very different from that of the first patient. **Accordingly**, a different treatment would be prescribed.

10　So the Chinese doctor, searching for and organizing signs and symptoms that a Western doctor might never **heed**, distinguishes the different patterns of disharmony where Western medicine perceives only one disease. The patterns of disharmony are similar to what the West calls diseases in that their discovery tells the physician how to prescribe treatment. But they are different from diseases because they cannot be isolated from the patient in whom they occur. To Western medicine, understanding an illness means uncovering a distinct entity that is separate from the patient's being; to Chinese medicine, understanding means perceiving the relationships between all the patient's signs and symptoms. When confronted by a patient with stomach pain, the Western physician must look beyond the screen of symptoms for an underlying pathological mechanism—a peptic ulcer in this case, but it could have been an infection or a tumor or a nervous disorder. A Chinese physician examining the same patient must discern a pattern of disharmony made up of the entire accumulation of symptoms and signs.

11　The Chinese method is thus holistic, based on the idea that no single part can be understood except in its relation to the whole. A symptom, therefore, is not traced back to a cause, but is looked at as a part of a totality. If a person has a symptom, Chinese medicine wants to know how the symptom fits into the patient's entire bodily pattern. A person who is well or "in harmony" has no distressing symptoms and expresses mental, physical, and spiritual balance. When that person is ill, the symptom is only one part of a complete bodily imbalance that can be seen in other aspects of his or her life and behavior. Understanding that overall pattern, with the symptom as part of it, is the challenge of Chinese medicine. The Chinese system is not less logical than the Western, just less analytical.

　　Reference: KAPTCHUK T J. The web that has no weaver: understanding Chinese medicine [M]. 2nd ed. New York: McGraw-Hill, 2000: 2-7.

New Words

extensive /ɪkˈstensɪv/	*a.*	large in amount or scale 大量的
clinician /klɪˈnɪʃn/	*n.*	a doctor having direct contact with patients rather than being involved with theoretical or laboratory studies 临床医生
sensibility /ˌsensɪˈbɪlɪti/	*n.*	the quality of being able to appreciate and respond to complex emotional or aesthetic influence 感悟(力)，感受(力)
perception /pəˈsepʃ(ə)n/	*n.*	the way in which sth. is regarded, understood, or interpreted 看法，理解，认识
perceptible /pəˈseptɪb(ə)l/	*a.*	(especially of a slight movement or change of state) able to be seen or noticed 可感觉(感受)到的，可理解的，可认识的
perceive /pəˈsiːv/	*vt.*	become aware or conscious of sth.; come to realize or understand 意识到；理解
endocrine /ˈendə(ʊ)kraɪn/	*a.*	relating to or denoting glands which secrete hormones or other products directly into the blood 内分泌(腺)的，激素的
pathological /ˌpæθəˈlɒdʒɪk(ə)l/	*a.*	relating to pathology 病理学的
pneumonia /njuːˈməʊnɪə/	*n.*	lung inflammation caused by bacterial or viral infection 肺炎
terminology /ˌtɜːmɪˈnɒlədʒi/	*n.*	the body of terms used with a particular technical application in a subject of study, theory, profession, etc. 术语
perspective /pəˈspektɪv/	*n.*	a particular attitude towards or way of regarding sth.; a point of view 看法，观点
stoke /stəʊk/	*vt.*	add coal or other solid fuel to (a fire) 拨旺火
extinguish /ɪkˈstɪŋgwɪʃ/	*vt.*	cause (a fire or light) to cease to burn or shine 熄灭(火)

笔记

17

rampage /ræmˈpeɪdʒ/	vi.	(especially of a large group of people) move through a place in a violent and uncontrollable manner 狂暴地乱冲
isolable /ˈaɪsələb(ə)l/	a.	being in the state of identifying sth. and examine or deal with it separately 孤立的
agent /ˈeɪdʒ(ə)nt/	n.	a substance that brings about a chemical or physical effect or causes a chemical reaction 任何能产生物理、化学或生物学效应的力、成分或物质；剂
ontologically /ˌɒntəˈlɒdʒɪk(ə)li/	ad.	connected with the branch of philosophy that deals with the nature of existence 存在论地；本体论地
circumscribe /ˈsɜːkəmskraɪb/	vt.	restrict (sth.) within limits 限制；限定
entity /ˈentɪti/	n.	a thing with distinct and independent existence 独立存在体；实体
privileged /ˈprɪvəlɪdʒd/	a.	having special rights or advantages that most people do not have 享有特权的；特许的，专用的
physician /fɪˈzɪʃ(ə)n/	n.	a person qualified to practice medicine, especially one who specializes in diagnosis and medical treatment as distinct from surgery 医生；(尤指)内科医生
precise /prɪˈsaɪs/	a.	marked by exactness and accuracy of expression or detail 明确的；确切的
self-contained /ˌself kənˈteɪnd/	a.	(of a thing) complete, or having all that is needed, in itself 自我完备的
quantifiable /ˌkwɒntɪˈfaɪəb(ə)l/	a.	able to be expressed or measured as a quantity 可量化的
accumulation /əˌkjuːmjʊˈleɪʃ(ə)n/	n.	a mass or quantity of sth. that has gradually gathered or been acquired 积累；累积量
scalpel /ˈskælp(ə)l/	n.	a knife with a small, sharp blade, as used by a surgeon 外科手术刀
physiological /ˌfɪziəˈlɒdʒɪk(ə)l/	a.	relating to the branch of biology that deals with the normal functions of living organisms and their parts 生理的
render /ˈrendə/	vt.	represent and depict artistically 表达；描绘

discern /dɪˈsɜːn/	vt.	recognize or find out 看出；理解，了解
organismic /ˌɔːgəˈnɪz(ə)mɪk/	a.	having the nature of, relating to or belonging to an organism (considered as a whole) 有机体的
synthetic /sɪnˈθetɪk/	a.	(of a substance) made by chemical synthesis, especially to imitate a natural product 综合的，合成的
configuration /kənˌfɪgəˈreɪʃ(ə)n/	n.	an arrangement of the parts of sth. or a group of things 结构，构型，组态
gastrointestinal /ˌgæstrəʊɪnˈtestɪn(ə)l/	a.	of or relating to the stomach and the intestines 胃肠的
endoscopy /enˈdɒskəpi/	n.	a procedure in which an instrument is introduced into the body to give a view of its internal parts 内镜检查术
fiberscope /ˈfaɪbəˌskəʊp/	n.	a fiber-optic device for viewing inaccessible internal structures, especially in the human body 纤维镜
peptic /ˈpeptɪk/	a.	of or relating to digestion, especially that in which pepsin（胃蛋白酶）is concerned 消化性的，（尤涉及）胃蛋白酶的
ulcer /ˈʌlsə/	n.	a sore area on the outside of the body or on the surface of an organ inside the body which is painful and may bleed or produce a poisonous substance 溃疡
palpation /pælˈpeɪʃ(ə)n/	n.	examining (a part of the body) by touch, especially for medical purposes 触诊，按诊
diminish /dɪˈmɪnɪʃ/	vi.	make or become less 减弱，减轻
compress /ˈkɒmpres/	n.	a cloth that is pressed onto a part of the body to stop the loss of blood, reduce pain, etc.（用于退热、止血等的）敷布
robust /rə(ʊ)ˈbʌst/	a.	strong and healthy; vigorous 健壮的；精力充沛的
constitution /ˌkɒnstɪˈtjuːʃ(ə)n/	n.	a person's physical state as regards vitality, health, and strength 体质；体格
complexion /kəmˈplekʃ(ə)n/	n.	the natural color, texture, and appearance of a person's skin, especially of the face 面色；肤色

笔记

assertive /əˈsəːtɪv/	a.	having or showing a confident and forceful personality 坚定而自信的
aggressive /əˈgresɪv/	a.	behaving or done in a determined and forceful way 积极进取的；有闯劲的；积极行动的
constipated /ˈkɒnstɪpeɪtɪd/	a.	unable to get rid of waste material from the bowels easily 患便秘的
urine /ˈjʊərɪn/	n.	a watery, typically yellowish fluid stored in the bladder and discharged through the urethra 尿
ashen /ˈæʃ(ə)n/	a.	(of a person's face) very pale with shock, fear, or illness 灰白色的
ruddy /ˈrʌdi/	a.	(of a person's face) having a healthy red color 红润的，血色好的
insomnia /ɪnˈsɒmnɪə/	n.	habitual sleeplessness; inability to sleep 失眠，失眠症
fidgety /ˈfɪdʒɪti/	a.	restless or uneasy 坐立不安的；烦躁的
moss /mɒs/	n.	a very small green or yellow plant without flowers that spreads over damp surfaces, rocks, trees, etc. 苔藓
accordingly /əˈkɔːdɪŋli/	ad.	as a result; therefore 于是；因此
heed /hiːd/	vt.	pay attention to; take notice of 注意，留心

Phrases and expressions

thought and practice	思想与实践
critical thinking	批判性思维
extensive clinical observation and testing	大量的临床观察和检验
be rooted in	根植于……，源于……
develop its own perception of health and illness	对健康与疾病形成独特的认识
neurological disorder	神经系统疾病，神经障碍，神经紊乱
endocrine disorder	内分泌紊乱
excess fire	实火
prevent liver wind from going to the head	防止肝风上扰
cultural affiliation	文化归属
agents of disease	病原体
zero in on	(使)对准……；全神贯注于(问题或主题)
underlying mechanism	潜在机制
in contrast	与此相反；相比之下

physiological and psychological	生理与心理的
pattern of disharmony	病证
diagnostic technique	诊断技术
precise cause	确切病因
cause and effect	因果(关系)
be secondary to	是次要的
symptoms and signs	症状与体征
provide the framework for treatment	提供治疗框架
from sb.'s perspective	从……的角度看
characterize...as...	把……的特征描述为……
damp heat affecting the spleen	湿热困脾
on the go	活跃,忙个不停
deficient yin affecting the stomach	胃阴虚(证)

Task One   Preview

1. Learn the following roots and affixes. Write out the Chinese meaning of the given words.

Roots/ Affixes	Meaning of roots/affixes	Words	Chinese meaning of the given words
anti-	against	antibiotic	_____
		antigen	_____
circum-	around	circumference	_____
		circumscribe	_____
crin (o)	secretion, the production of a substance	endocrine	_____
		endocrinology	_____
dis-	lack of; not	disease	_____
		disharmony	_____
endo-	within	endomembrane	_____
		endoscope	_____
gastr (o)	stomach	gastritis	_____
		gastrointestinal	_____
-ia	disease; pathological or abnormal condition	leukemia	_____
		pneumonia	_____
in-	not; the opposite or lack of sth.	insignificant	_____
		insensible	_____
per-	through	permanent	_____
		perspective	_____

笔记

physi (o)-	relating to natural forces or function	physical	_____
		physiological	_____
pneum (o)	air, lung breathing	pneumology	_____
		pneumonia	_____
press	press	compress	_____
		oppression	_____
-scope	instrument	endoscope	_____
		fiberscope	_____
sens-	feel	sensibility	_____
		sensor	_____
sol	alone	isolate	_____
		solo	_____
somn (i)	sleep	insomnia	_____
		somnambulate	_____
tens	stretch	extensive	_____
		intensive	_____
termin	limit	determine	_____
		terminology	_____

2. Write down the questions you would like to ask or discuss about the text.

_____

_____

_____

Task Two Vocabulary

Choose the word or phrase that can best complete the statements.

1) Many factors contribute to the onset（发病）of a disease, including _____ ones such as six evils, physical damage or trauma, metal wounds or insect bite.

    A. infectious   B. endogenous   C. exogenous   D. traumatic

2) According to World Health Organization, "traditional medicine refers to health practices, approaches, knowledge and beliefs _____ plant, animal and mineral based medicines, spiritual therapies, manual techniques and exercises, _____ singularly or in combination to treat, diagnose and prevent illnesses or maintain well-being."

    A. incorporating; applying   B. incorporated; applied

    C. incorporating; applied   D. incorporated; applying

3) Health exists if adequate qi, blood and body fluids are _____ equitably and smoothly.

    A. distributed   B. flowed   C. contained   D. balanced

4) How the human body is _____ and explained varies in the East and the West, as do the methods used to treat illness.

    A. treated   B. cured   C. defined   D. perceived

5) Illness is attributed to imbalance or interruption of qi. Ancient practices such as acupuncture, qigong, and the use of various herbs are claimed to _____ balance.

    A. keep   B. maintain   C. lose   D. restore

6) The patients who received acupuncture also fell asleep faster, were less _____ at night, and were less stressed.

    A. arisen   B. aroused   C. risen   D. rosin

7) By the opposition of yin and yang, we mean all things and phenomena in the natural world contain the two _____ components.

    A. counterpart   B. counterbalance   C. opponent   D. opposite

8) The conditions claimed to respond to acupuncture include chronic pain (neck and back pain, migraine headaches), acute injury-related pain (strains, muscle and ligament tears), and _____ problems (indigestion, ulcers, constipation, diarrhea).

    A. gastrointestinal   B. stomach

    C. belly   D. intestinal

9) In this article we _____ the research and commentary literature on the current and emerging relationship between biomedicine and traditional medicine.

    A. conduct   B. do   C. explore   D. inquire

10) There are a number of ways in which a/an _____ mainstream health care system may operate, with many challenges posed by trying to meld these two fundamentally different paradigms of health care.

    A. comprehensive   B. combining   C. integrated   D. united

11) Complementary and alternative medical therapies including yoga are commonly used in children _____ with attention deficit hyperactivity disorder, but little is known about the efficacy of these therapies.

    A. diagnosis   B. diagnosed   C. diagnosing   D. to diagnose

12) The theoretical _____ must demonstrate an understanding of theories and concepts that are relevant to the topic of your research paper and that relate to the broader areas of knowledge being considered.

    A. knowledge   B. methodology   C. structure   D. framework

13) *Zangxiang* theory pays more attention to the synthetic _____ of the holistic functions of the body and is more sophisticated in cognizing the intrinsic nature of life from the external _____.

    A. manifestations; manifestations   B. indications; indications

    C. signs; signs   D. symptoms; symptoms

14) Insufficient qi production caused by blood deficiency is manifested as pale or sallow (蜡黄色) _____, lassitude (困乏), vertigo (眩晕), palpitation (心悸), etc.

    A. face   B. color   C. complexion   D. skin

15) Interest in TCM was sparked in the United States in the early 1970s when *New York Times* reporter James Reston experienced a/an _____ appendicitis (阑尾炎) attack while in China.

A. urgent　　　　　B. acute　　　　　C. chronic　　　　　D. emergent

Task Three　Translation

Translate the following expressions into English.

1) 卫气营血　　　　　　　　　2) 草药

3) 食疗　　　　　　　　　　　4) 临床观察与实践

5) 道家学派　　　　　　　　　6) 中医整体观

7) 辨证　　　　　　　　　　　8) 治疗八法

9) 吐法　　　　　　　　　　　10) 下法

11) 消法　　　　　　　　　　12) 天人相应

13) 诊断与治疗　　　　　　　14) 传统的师承制

15) 致病因素　　　　　　　　16) 中药学，中药

17) 神经疾病　　　　　　　　18) 内分泌疾病

19) 实火　　　　　　　　　　20) 生理与心理的

笔记

PART Ⅲ　TRANSLATION AND WRITING

How to Introduce Traditional Chinese Medicine

Although traditional Chinese medicine (TCM) has a history of more than two thousand years, it became known to Westerners only a few decades ago. Very different from Western medicine, TCM has its unique value to contribute to the human well-being. Statistics indicate that TCM is gaining increasing popularity in the world. As a result, we are obliged to learn to introduce some important aspects about TCM, for instance, its connotation (内涵), its classic works, its diagnosis and treatment as well as its uniqueness as a medical system. A better understanding of TCM is perhaps based on a comparison and contrast with Western medicine. We may take the following aspects into consideration: different perception of health, disease, symptom, approaches of treatment, as well as the underlying philosophy, etc.

The following sentences or expressions are commonly used to introduce TCM.

1) Taken as a whole, TCM more precisely refers to a shared experience of medical knowledge of all ethnic groups in China.

从整体上看,更准确地说,中医是中国各民族医学知识的通称。

2) Different from Western medicine that focuses on diseases, TCM was established on a holistic harmony between man and nature for thousands of years.

中医不同于西医。西医聚焦于疾病,而有几千年历史的中医是建立在人与自然和谐统一的整体观上。

3) TCM has not only withstood the tests of time, but has passed the tests of modern medicine.

中医不仅经受了时间的洗礼,还经受了现代医学的挑战。

4) Is TCM science or superstition? The documented effectiveness of TCM practices speaks for itself. We'll let you decide.

中医是科学还是迷信?文献中关于中医疗效的记载就是最好的回答。你可以自己做出判断。

5) As one of the world's ancient medical sciences, TCM with its distinctive concepts and methods is believed to compensate for the deficiencies of Western medicine, and is gaining global popularity.

作为世界古代医学之一,中医学以其独特的理念与方法弥补了西医的不足,逐渐受到全球欢迎。

6) The gist of *Huangdi's Inner Canon of Medicine* is that human existence is like a microcosm in the infinite universe; therefore, people must achieve constant harmony with the law of nature and the changing seasons.

《黄帝内经》的核心观点是,人就像存在于广袤无垠的宇宙中的一个微观世界,因此人必须道法自然,遵循四季的变化,不断获取调适的状态。

7) The yin-yang doctrine and the theory of the five phases in *Huangdi's Inner Canon*

of Medicine are not only the foundation for the established medicine system of TCM, but also an expression of Confucian sociopolitical ideas and theory.

《黄帝内经》中的阴阳学说与五行学说不仅是中医理论体系的基础,也是儒家社会政治思想和理论的体现。

8) TCM thinks of qi as life and that life and medicine are one. Western medicine believes that humans can control nature, and has its focus on external causes of maladies.

中医认为气乃生命之源,生命和医药是一个整体。西医则认为人类可以控制自然,并关注疾病的外因。

9) Diagnosis in TCM may appear to be simply a grouping of symptoms, but the elegance of TCM is that a diagnosis automatically indicates a treatment strategy.

表面上看,中医诊断只是简单地把症状进行分类,但中医的美妙之处就在于确定诊断的同时治疗方案也随之确定。

10) TCM is a great treasure house and efforts should be made to explore them and raise them to a higher level.

中医药学是一个伟大的宝库,应当努力发掘,加以提高。

11) In TCM, health is a state of well-being where the body is in balance with and adaptive to the environment. Western doctors consider health to be the absence of disease, pain or defect.

中医认为健康是一种身体调适且适应环境的良好状态。西医认为健康就是无病、无痛或没有缺损。

12) To TCM practitioners, disease is caused by an imbalance of the vital force of the body and stems from multiple causes, while Westerners think of it as a defect of tissue or structure of the organism with a single cause.

在中医看来,疾病源于人体机能的失衡,且病因多样;而西方人则认为疾病是源于机体组织或结构的缺损,且病因单一。

13) One of the key differences is the approach. The approach with Western medicine is deductive and analytical, while TCM uses an inductive and synthetic approach.

关键的不同之处在于方法。西医的方法是演绎和分析,而中医采用归纳和综合的方法。

14) Symptoms, in TCM view, are messages from the body about its state of balance or vitality and should be listened to carefully. To the Western doctor, symptoms are signs of the disease or defect and should be reduced or eliminated.

在中医看来,症状是机体发出的有关其平衡或活力状态的信息,应该仔细倾听。对西医而言,症状是疾病或缺损的表现,应当减少或消除。

15) We need both TCM and Western medicine. The sooner we integrate both into a universal approach to healing and treatment, the healthier and wiser we will all be.

我们需要中医,也需要西医。我们越快整合二者为一种普适方法来治病疗伤,就会越来越健康和明智。

笔记

Sample

TCM: An Individualized Approach

When a TCM doctor exams a patient, he or she will ask a series of questions. 1) Instead of trying to narrow down the cause of a symptom to one specific source, the doctor of TCM, however, would try to find out the sources for the symptom as many as possible by uncovering all of the physiological circumstances that could be surrounding it.

2) A TCM doctor would make a diagnosis unique to this individual patient based on these characteristics. Even though the endoscopic exam might reveal a peptic ulcer, this patient would not be seen as having the same problem as any other patient with a peptic ulcer. A solitary lesion might appear in the antral portion of his stomach, but the conditions surrounding its appearance would be unique to him.

Theoretically, three different patients with solitary lesions on their stomachs could receive three entirely different diagnoses. A TCM doctor might diagnose damp heat affecting the spleen in one, deficient yin affecting the stomach in another, and disharmony between the liver and the spleen in the third.

3) From the standpoint of Western medicine, disease can be separated from the patient. It is something that the patient has. Thus, any number of patients can also have the disease and be treated in a similar manner. In TCM, however, disease is not viewed as something that a patient has. It is something that the patient is. 4) Disease, from the Chinese point of view, is an imbalance in the patient's being. There is no isolated, self-contained, separate entity called "disease". There is only a whole person whose body functions may be balanced or imbalanced, harmonious or disharmonious. 5) Understanding the nature of the imbalance is the goal of diagnosis, while restoring balance is the focus of treatment.

Task One   Translation

Translate the underlined parts in the above sample into Chinese.

1) _____

_____

2) _____

_____

3) _____

_____

4) _____

_____

5) _____

_____

Task Two   Writing

Write a 200-word composition to introduce traditional Chinese medicine. Try to use

27

as many sentence patterns as possible in PART Ⅲ. Alternatively, you may work in pairs on the given topic, search the information on the internet, write the composition and then present it to the class.

_____

_____

_____

PART IV   REFLECTION

Some TCM university/college students do not think they should be required to learn English, let alone learn TCM English. They think they can hire a translator if they need to communicate with people in other cultures. Others maintain that learning English is particularly essential for the sake of disseminating TCM culture since TCM is gaining increasing popularity across the globe.

Interview a couple of teachers and students in your university/college, and ask the following questions:

1) Is it important for TCM university/college students to learn English?

2) What role does English language play in the dissemination of TCM?

Unit 2

Philosophies and Concepts of Traditional Chinese Medicine

LEARNING OUTCOMES

This unit offers you opportunities to:

- **explain** briefly the theories of yin-yang and five phases
- **give** examples to illustrate functions of the heart in traditional Chinese medicine (TCM)
- **use** the terms related to philosophies and concepts of TCM
- **define** a Chinese medical term
- **reflect on** standardizing translation of TCM terms

PART I   LISTENING AND SPEAKING

Before you listen

In this section you will hear a short passage entitled "Key Concepts of Traditional Chinese Medicine". The following words and phrases may be of help.

duality /djuːˈælɪti/	*n.*	二元性
highlight /ˈhaɪlaɪt/	*vt.*	强调,突出
impermanence /ɪmˈpɜːmənəns/	*n.*	暂时,无常
fluidity /fluːˈɪdɪti/	*n.*	流动性;不稳定
interaction /ˌɪntərˈækʃ(ə)n/	*n.*	相互作用
generate /ˈdʒenəreɪt/	*vt.*	产生,引起
vein /veɪn/	*n.*	静脉,脉
immunity /ɪˈmjuːnɪti/	*n.*	免疫力
containment /kənˈteɪnm(ə)nt/	*n.*	控制;抑制
transformation /ˌtrænsfəˈmeɪʃ(ə)n/	*n.*	转化
revolve round		围绕
life force		生命力
life process		生命过程

While you listen

Listen to the passage carefully and fill in each of the blanks marked from 1) to 10) according to what you have heard.

Key Concepts of Traditional Chinese Medicine

Traditional Chinese medicine (TCM) is a highly complex topic based on a million 1)_____. However, there are a few key philosophies around which all TCM 2)_____. The most central concept of all is that of yin and yang, an idea which 3)_____ in the 16th century B.C. Yin and yang represent a universal balance and duality present in all things, from the movement of the stars and planets to bodily functions. Yin is characterized by dark, cold and damp, whereas yang is characterized by light, heat and dryness. In TCM maintaining a 4)_____ relationship between yin and yang within the body is of uttermost importance. Another highly important concept is known as *wuxing* or the five phases. Where yin and yang may be classified as the concepts of balance, *wuxing* highlights the 5)_____ and fluidity of all things. *Wuxing* proposes that there are five elemental 6)_____ to everything: wood, fire, earth, metal and water. And

ER-2-1
Listening
practice

笔记

31

there are two types of interactions between these states: 7)_____ interactions and restricting interactions. In TCM, the *wuxing* theory explains many interactions within the body, especially relationships between different organs. A third concept is that of qi, commonly referred to as 8)_____ or energy. In TCM, there are two types of qi: qi that flows in the veins and qi that exists in the 9)_____ and tissue. And all qi plays five roles: fulfillment of life processes, providing warmth, providing 10)_____, containment and transformation.

After you listen

Please discuss with your partner the following questions and give your presentation to the class.

1) What are the interactions that *wuxing* explains between different organs?
2) What are the functions of qi?

PART II   READING

Text A

The Theory of Yin and Yang

1   The theory of yin and yang, derived from age-long observation of nature, describes the way phenomena naturally group in pairs of opposites—heaven and earth, sun and moon, day and night, summer and winter, male and female, up and down, inside and outside, movement and **stasis**. These pairs of opposites are also mutual **complements**. Chapter 5 of *Su Wen* (*Plain Questions*)① states: "Yin and yang are the law of heaven and earth."

The basic principles of yin-yang theory

2   All phenomena in the universe may be **ascribed** to yin and yang. Each individual phenomenon possesses both a yin and a yang aspect. Yin and yang are natural complements in the sense that they depend upon and **counterbalance** each other. Further, they are mutually **convertible**, since either may change into its complement.

Yin and yang as the fundamental categories of all phenomena

3   In medicine, the concepts of yin and yang are generally used to categorize both **anatomic** parts and physiologic functions. For example, the back is yang and the **abdomen** is yin; the six *fu*-organs② are yang and the five *zang*-organs③ are yin; qi is yang and blood is yin; **agitation** is yang and **moderation** is yin. Similarly, diseases may be categorized according to yin and yang. For example, exterior, **excess** and heat disorders are yang, while interior, **deficiency**, and cold disorders are yin. Pulses may similarly be categorized: floating, rapid, and **slippery** pulses are yang, while deep, slow, and rough pulses are yin.

Yin-yang analysis of physiologic activity

4   Yin and yang provide a general method of analyzing the functions of the human body. These are seen in terms of four categories of movement: **upbearing**, **downbearing**, exit, and entry.④ Upbearing and exit are yang, while downbearing and entry are yin. These movements serve to explain the interactions between blood and qi, and the organs and meridians.

5   Physiologic processes are explained in terms of the natural **flux** of yin and yang. *Su Wen* states: "Clear yang exits from the upper **portals**,⑤ while **turbid** yin exits from the lower portals; clear yang **effuses** (exits) through the **striations**, while turbid yin goes through (enters) the five *zang*-organs; clear yang fills the limbs, whereas turbid yin passes

---

① *Su Wen* (*Plain Questions*):《素问》,又译为 *Basic Questions* 或 *Elementary Questions*。
② six *fu*-organs: 六腑,也可译为 six bowels。
③ five *zang*-organs: 五脏,也可译为 five viscera。
④ upbearing, downbearing, exit, and entry: 升降出入,也可译为 upward, downward, inward and outward movement 或 ascending, descending, exiting and entering。
⑤ portal: 孔窍,也常译为 orifice。

笔记

through the six *fu*-organs."

6   This explains how yang, the clear light qi of the body, ascends up to and out of the portals, passing outward to the surface of the skin and strengthening the limbs, and how yin, the heavy turbid qi of the body, flows in the interior, its waste products being **discharged** through the **anus** and the **urethra**.① The four movements are considered to be interdependent and mutually supporting. Thus *Su Wen* states: "Yin is in the inner body and protects yang; yang is in the outer body and moves yin."

Yin-yang analysis of pathologic change

7   In medicine, **morbidity** is explained in terms of yin-yang imbalance. Both pathogenic and healthy qi can be analyzed in terms of yin and yang. There are both yin and yang **pathogens**. Yin pathogens cause a **surfeit** of yin, which manifests as a cold pattern; yang pathogens produce a surfeit of yang in the body characterized by excess heat pattern. The "healthy qi", the body's health-maintaining forces, comprise two aspects, yang qi and yin fluid. Yang-qi deficiency is characterized by deficiency-cold patterns, whereas yin-fluid deficiency is characterized by deficiency-heat patterns. A vast number of diseases can be summed up in the following four phrases: When yin **prevails**, there is cold; when yang prevails, there is heat. When yang is deficient, there is cold; when yin is deficient, there is heat.

8   The cause of these conditions is imbalance—surfeits or deficits②—of either yin or yang.

General parameters of diagnosis

9   Imbalance of yin and yang accounts for the emergence and development of a disease. The essential nature of any disease may be analyzed in terms of yin and yang, despite the infinite number of possible clinical manifestations. Yin and yang form the basic **parameters** of eight parameter pattern differentiation:③ exterior, heat, and excess disorders being yang; interior, cold and deficiency disorders being yin. *Su Wen* states: "Proper diagnosis involves inspecting the complexion and feeling the pulse and first differentiating yin and yang."

Treatment and medicinal use

10   Because a surfeit of yin or yang is the primary cause of any disease, treatment must involve restoring the balance by reducing excess and supplying insufficiency.

11   The nature and effect of herbal medicinals may also be classified according to yin and yang. For example, cold, cool, rich, and moist agents are yin, whereas warm, hot, dry, and fierce agents are yang. Agents **pungent** and sweet in taste are yang, while those that are salty, bitter, sour or **astringent**④ in taste are yin. Agents that upbear and effuse are yang in nature, and agents that contract and astringe are yin.

---

① anus and urethra: 肛门和尿道，属于中医所称的"二阴"。
② surfeits or deficits: 盛或衰。
③ eight parameter pattern differentiation: 八纲辨证，也可译为 pattern differentiation according to eight principles。
④ astringent: 涩的；中药五味是酸、苦、甘、辛、咸，对应地翻译为 sour, bitter, sweet, acrid/pungent, and salty。

12   Therefore, in diagnosis and treatment, it is necessary to identify yin-yang surfeits and deficits among the complex array of symptoms and determine the nature of the treatment. Agents must also be selected and used to make an appropriate **synthesis** of their yin and yang qualities. This means that a pattern due to a surfeit of yin or yang is one of excess, and according to the principle of reducing excess, is treated by the method of **drainage**[①]. A pattern essentially the result of a deficit of either yin or yang is one of deficiency, and in accordance with the principle of supplying insufficiency, is treated by the method of **supplementation**. If yin is in surfeit, the problem is one of excess-cold, for which pungent yang agents warm in nature should be used to **dissipate** the cold. If yang is in surfeit, the pattern is one of excess-heat, requiring cold, bitter heat drainers,[②] which are yin in nature. If the pattern **stems** from an insufficiency of yin, yin supplementing agents with a cooling and moistening effect are **prescribed** to nourish blood and fluids.[③] Conditions stemming from a yang deficit manifest themselves as deficiency-cold, and are treated with yang medicinals, warm or hot agents, to warm and supplement yang qi.

Reference: WISEMAN N, ELLIS A. The fundamentals of Chinese medicine [M]. Brookline, Massachusetts: Paradigm Publications, 1996: 1-7.

New words

stasis /'steɪsɪs/	n.	a situation in which there is no change or development 静止
complement /'kɒmplɪm(ə)nt/	n.	a thing that contributes extra features to sth. else in such a way as to improve or emphasize its quality 补足物
ascribe /ə'skraɪb/	vi.	regard sth. as being due to (a cause) 把……归于
counterbalance /'kaʊntə,bæl(ə)ns/	vt.	neutralize or cancel by exerting an opposite influence 抵消
convertible /kən'vɜːtɪb (ə)l/	a.	able to be changed in form, function, or character 可改变的;可变换的
anatomic /,ænə'tɒmik/	a.	relating to bodily structure 解剖的
abdomen /'æbdəmən/	n.	the part of the body of a vertebrate containing the digestive and reproductive organs; the belly 腹部
agitation /,ædʒɪ'teɪʃ(ə)n/	n.	a state of anxiety or nervous excitement 躁动

---

① drainage: 常表示"排空",此处表示"泻"。
② cold, bitter heat drainers: 意为"苦寒的泻热药"。
③ nourish blood and fluids: 可理解为"补养津血"。

moderation /ˌmɔdəˈreɪʃ(ə)n/	n.	the avoidance of excess or extremes, especially in one's behavior or political opinions 温和,适度
excess /ɪkˈses/	n.	an amount of sth. that is more than necessary, permitted, or desirable 超过
deficiency /dɪˈfɪʃ(ə)nsi/	n.	a lack of shortage 缺乏,不足
slippery /ˈslɪp(ə)ri/	a.	(of a surface or an object) difficult to hold firmly or stand on because it is smooth, wet, or slimy 滑的
upbearing /ʌpˈbeərɪŋ/	n.	turning and proceeding in an upward direction 向上
downbearing /daʊnˈbeərɪŋ/	n.	turning and proceeding in a downward direction 向下
flux /flʌks/	n.	the action or process of flowing or flowing out 流量,流出
portal /ˈpɔːt(ə)l/	n.	a doorway, gate, or other entrance, especially a large and imposing one 大门,入口
turbid /ˈtəːbɪd/	a.	cloudy, opaque, or thick with suspended matter 浑浊的
effuse /ɪˈfjuːs/	vt.	give off (a liquid, light, smell, or quality) 涌出,流出
striation /straɪˈeɪʃ(ə)n/	n.	the state marked with striae 纹理
discharge /dɪsˈtʃɑːdʒ/	v.	allow (a liquid, gas, or other substance) to flow out from where it has been confined 排放
anus /ˈeɪnəs/	n.	the opening at the end of the alimentary canal through which solid waste matter leaves the body 肛门
urethra /juˈriːθrə/	n.	the duct by which urine is conveyed out of the body from the bladder, and which in male vertebrates also conveys semen 尿道
morbidity /mɔːˈbɪdɪti/	n.	the condition of being diseased 病态;发病
pathogen /ˈpæθədʒ(ə)n/	n.	a bacterium, virus, or other microorganism that can cause disease 病原体
surfeit /ˈsəːfɪt/	n.	an excessive amount of sth. 过度
prevail /prɪˈveɪl/	vi.	prove more powerful or superior 战胜,占上风

parameter /pəˈræmɪtə/	n.	a numerical or other measurable factor forming one of a set that defines a system or sets the conditions of its operation 参数
medicinal /məˈdɪsɪn(ə)l/	a.	(of a substance or plant) having healing properties 医学的,药用的
	n.	a medicinal substance 药品
pungent /ˈpʌn(d)ʒ(ə)nt/	a.	having a sharply strong taste or smell 辛辣的
astringent /əˈstrɪn(d)ʒ(ə)nt/	a.	causing the contraction of skin cells and other body tissues 收涩的
synthesis /ˈsɪnθɪsɪs/	n.	the combination of components or elements to form a connected whole 综合,合成
drainage /ˈdreɪnɪdʒ/	n.	the action or process of draining sth. 排水
supplementation /ˌsʌplɪmenˈteɪʃ(ə)n/	n.	a thing added to sth. else in order to complete or enhance it 增补
dissipate /ˈdɪsɪpeɪt/	vt.	disperse or scatter 驱散
stem /stem/	vi.	originate in or be caused by 源于
prescribe /prɪˈskraɪb/	vt.	(of a medical practitioner) advise and authorize the use of (a medicine or treatment) for someone, especially in writing 开处方

Phrases and expressions

derive from	源于;衍生于
be ascribed to	归结于
clear yang	清阳
upper portals	上窍
turbid yin	浊阴
five *zang*-organs	五脏
six *fu*-organs	六腑
anus and the urethra	二阴
yin-yang imbalance	阴阳失调
pathogenic and healthy qi	邪气和正气
yin and yang pathogens	阴邪和阳邪
account for	对……负有责任;导致;(比例)占
inspect the complexion	望面色
feel the pulse	把脉

stem from	源于;造成;基于
nourish blood	养血
warm and supplement yang qi	温补阳气

Task One   Preview

1. Learn the following roots and affixes. Write out the Chinese meaning of the given words.

Roots/ Affixes	Meaning of roots/affixes	Words	Chinese meaning of the given words
abdomin (o)	abdomen	abdominal	_____
		abdominothoracic	_____
acu-	needle	acupoint	_____
		acupuncture	_____
ana-	apart	analysis	_____
		anatomy	_____
-asthenia	weakness	pulmonasthenia	_____
		myasthenia	_____
cide	kill	pesticide	_____
		suicide	_____
counter-	against; opposite	counteraction	_____
		counterbalance	_____
cry (o)	cold	cryogen	_____
		cryopreservation	_____
dual	double	duality	_____
		dualism	_____
fus	pour	effuse	_____
		infuse	_____
-genic	causing	carcinogenic	_____
		mutagenic	_____
-meter	instrument for measuring	chronometer	_____
		thermometer	_____
hepa/hepat	liver	hepatic	_____
		hepatitis	_____
neo-	new	neonatal	_____
		neoplasm	_____
pan-	all, wide	pancarditis	_____
		pandemic	_____

string	tighten	astringent	_____
		constringent	_____
supra-	upper	supraclavicular	_____
		suprarenal	_____
syn	join	syndrome	_____
		synergy	_____
therm (o)	heat, temperature	thermoplegia	_____
		thermolysis	_____

2. Write down the questions you would like to ask or discuss about the text.

_____

_____

_____

Task Two   Speaking

1. Answer the following questions according to the text.

1) How did the yin-yang theory come into being?

2) What are the basic principles of the yin-yang theory illustrated in this article?

3) What can the yin-yang theory be used to do in TCM?

4) In what ways could yang qi go outwards and strengthen the limbs?

5) Why can qi and blood interact with each other?

6) How is morbidity explained by the yin-yang theory?

7) What is the first principle in the eight parameter pattern differentiation?

8) How are the nature and the taste of herbs classified according to yin and yang?

2. Work in pairs or groups and exchange views on the following passage.

Chinese Medicine Today:

Issues for Research, Education and Practice in the West

The transmission of Chinese medicine historically, and to countries outside China, has largely been possible due to the textual legacy that has recorded its conceptual and therapeutic developments. Today, Chinese- and Western-generated TCM textbooks are the main route of Chinese medicine transmission globally. During the middle of the twentieth century, the architects of TCM consolidated Chinese medicine's diverse and disparate (完全不同的) currents and systematized Chinese medical theory-practice. TCM textbooks were created to present structured frameworks for the learning and application of traditional medical theories. The new textbooks revised premodern conceptual models and treatment methods to suit the contemporary reader and today's bioscientific medical culture. These developments have raised questions concerning the modernization of Chinese medicine and the relevance of its traditional methods, and the gulf that has developed between Chinese medicine's "basic theory" and its clinical applications.

When the Chinese decided to modernize and scientize their national medicine, their revisions included a number of projects aimed at formulating theoretical principles and standardizing therapeutic content. For instance, pattern differentiation was redefined to encompass conflicting premodern diagnostic methods. The great success of the new pattern differentiation model was its capacity to also incorporate biomedical disease categories into TCM diagnostic analysis. To facilitate the newly developed centralized teaching curriculum, disease and pattern analysis had to be standardized, as did therapeutic principles, medicinal actions, acupoint features, locations, methods and a raft（大量）of related terms.

On the positive side, standardizing and scientizing Chinese medicine content and categories created disease classification structures and treatment strategies with clear lines of separation. Standardized terms and diagnostic criteria gave the discipline（学科）a firm foundation for learning and promised to improve the inter-examiner reliability of Chinese medicine practice and research. More recently, the moves to standardize the English translation of Chinese medical terminology have alerted many Westerners to the breadth and complexity of its technical language.

Chinese medical terms are used in different ways depending on the historical context, so standardizing the translation of terms is not without problems. While source-based translations attempt to preserve historical contexts and connections, bioscientific translations endeavor to align premodern concepts with contemporary scientific understanding. Standardized biomedical translations of Chinese terms in particular decouple（割裂，分裂）contextual meanings from clinical methods, erase thousands of years of diversity and remove some of the tradition's inbuilt flexibility. Moreover, when guided by a bioscientific agenda the translation of traditional terms leads to a sense that TCM is essentially similar to bioscientific medicine.

The biomedicalization of terms is one example of how modernization has affected the transmission of Chinese medicine as a distinct field of medicine. Medical anthropologists（人类学家）have explored the vulnerability（弱点，脆弱）of traditional medical systems to the political hegemony（霸权）of biomedicine. For example, the global dominance and momentum（势头）of scientific medicine means that the biomedicine-and-state "body politic" defines efficacy and how to measure it. Consequently, the integration of Chinese medicine and biomedicine is in reality a one-sided process that biomedicalizes health care.

Advocates of scientization argue that it must be possible to utilize and test Chinese medicine from within a biomedical framework, and if scientization means removing Chinese medicine's traditional principles and concepts then surely it could be made more efficient and more effective in the process. For contemporary health care professionals and researchers this is a persuasive option. To understand why, we only have to consider Chinese medicine's conservative historical legacy, its complex and disparate currents, its apparent neglect of physical structures and mechanisms, its incompatible assumptions and methodological dissonance（不一致）with biomedicine and our problems with access to premodern sources.

40

Reference: GARVEY M. Chinese medicine today: issues for research, education and practice in the West [J]. Australian journal of acupuncture & Chinese medicine, 2013, 8 (1):28–34.

Topic for discussion: What are the pros and cons of standardizing and scientizing TCM?

Task Three   Vocabulary

1. Match up each word in Column A with its appropriate definition from Column B.

Column A	Column B
1) stasis	a. intestine
2) agitation	b. belly
3) pathogen	c. the internal organs in the main cavities of the body
4) bowel	d. a drug or chemical capable of eliciting a biological response
5) anatomic	e. a stoppage of flow of a body fluid
6) viscera	f. opening at the end of the alimentary canal through which solid waste matter leaves the body
7) urethra	g. a state of anxiety or nervous excitement
8) abdomen	h. relating to bodily structure
9) anus	i. the duct by which urine is conveyed out of the body from the bladder
10) prescribe	j. the condition of being diseased
11) morbidity	k. a bacterium, virus, or other microorganism that can cause disease
12) agent	l. advise and authorize the use of (a medicine or treatment) for someone

2. Fill in the blanks with the words given below. Change the form where necessary.

phase	manifestation	pathogen	bowel	urine
stasis	organism	symptom	urethra	viscera
balance	pungent	agent	meridian	bitter

Basic Concepts of TCM

In TCM, yin refers largely to the material aspects of the 1)_____ and yang to functions. There is a circulation of qi (energy) and blood. The organs work together by regulating and preserving qi and blood through the so-called 2)_____ and collaterals. Disease occurs after a disturbance in yin-yang or flow of qi or blood, or disharmony in the organs caused by 3)_____ (e.g. sadness, joy, lifestyle) and climatic factors (dampness, heat, cold). Treatment aims to expel or suppress the cause and restore 4)_____.

Imbalance is assessed by four traditional examination methods: looking, listening and smelling, asking, and palpation. Observations of the pulse, face, tongue, 5) _____ and stool provide essential information. The diagnosis is derived with theories such as the eight diagnostic principles to differentiate between yin-yang, interior-exterior, deficiency-excess, and cold-heat, the five 6) _____ theory to assess the relations between organs and functions, and the 7) _____ manifestation theory to establish the disease location.

The diagnosis that guides treatment is called *zheng*, a temporary state at one time and which is like a syndrome defined by 8) _____ and signs. The same disease in Western medicine can 9) _____ in different *zheng*s and vice versa. Thus, treatment in the same patient varies over time and the same disease can be treated differently. For example, kidney yin deficiency as a *zheng* has three components: kidney, yin, and deficiency. Other examples include preponderant liver yang, flaring up of heart fire, and spleen-stomach dampness-heat. For each or a combination of the components, there are specific herbs or treatments. For example, 10) _____ herbs are cool in nature and can be used to treat heat-ridden diseases. TCM can make diagnoses and treat patients without needing a scientific understanding of cause and pathogenesis.

Reference: TANG J L, LIU B Y, MA K W. Traditional Chinese medicine [J]. The lancet, 372 (9654): 1938–1940. DOI: http://dx.doi.org/10.1016/S0140-6736 (08)61354-9.

Task Four   Translation

1. Study the following sentences and pay attention to the underlined parts.

1) The theory of yin and yang, <u>derived from</u> age-long observation of nature, describes the way phenomena naturally group in pairs of opposites. (para. 1)

2) All phenomena in the universe may <u>be ascribed to</u> yin and yang. (para. 2)

3) These are seen <u>in terms of</u> four categories of movement: upbearing, downbearing, exit, and entry. (para. 4)

4) These movements <u>serve to</u> explain the interactions between blood and qi, and the organs and meridians. (para. 4)

5) Imbalance of yin and yang <u>accounts for</u> the emergence and development of disease. (para. 9)

6) If the pattern <u>stems from</u> an insufficiency of yin, yin supplementing agents with a cooling and moistening effect <u>are prescribed</u> to nourish blood and fluids. (para. 12)

2. Translate the following sentences into English.

1) 食管（esophageal）疾病可以是先天性的，也可以是后天获得的。

2) “肥胖（obesity）流行病”的发生在很大程度上归因于体育活动的减少和食物质量、饮食习惯的差异。

3) 疫苗（vaccine）是众多延长人类寿命花费中最好的方式之一。

4) 在这方面,这一工具将起到减少婴幼儿死亡和患病的作用。

5) 同样的缺陷导致了大多数常见的人类双色(dichromatic)色盲症。

6) 感冒可由风寒、风热或体虚引起,所以医生会用不同的方剂治疗。

Text B

Heart

1　The heart is said to be the most important of all the *zang–fu* organs. It is sometimes called the "great governor of the five *zang* and six *fu* organs". Its main functions are to govern blood and vessels, and to store *shen* (spirit). The heart opens into the tongue and controls sweat.

Governing blood and vessels

2　By the phrase "the heart governs the blood and vessels of the body," *Su Wen* (*Basic Questions*) emphasizes that all the blood and vessels of the body are **subordinate** to the heart. Although blood is produced from the essence of grain and water **assimilated** by the stomach and spleen, it is the heart that ensures constant circulation of blood, maintaining the supply of **nourishment** to the whole body. Thus *Su Wen* states: "All blood is subordinate to the heart," and "The vessels are the house of blood."

3　Just as in Western scientific views, if the functioning of the heart is poor, supply of blood to the tissues is deficient, i.e., heart blood deficiency—which can cause cold **extremities**.

4　Although the human constitution is said to be determined by the kidney essence, it is also partly related to the heart and blood. If the heart is strong and the supply of blood in the body is plentiful, the person will be strong.

Storing *shen* (spirit)

5　"The heart stores the spirit" is the same in meaning as "the heart governs the spirit." Here, "spirit" refers to the clarity of the **consciousness** and strength of mental faculties. It encompasses emotional, mental, and spiritual aspects of the whole body; in this sense it plays an important role in all the organs' functions—especially the yin organs. In Western physiology, both consciousness and mental activity are considered functions of the brain, but in Chinese medicine their different aspects are variously attributed to the organs. The heart is considered particularly important in this context. If the heart fulfills its functions normally and blood and qi are abundant, the spirit-mind is lucid, making the individual alert and responsive to the environment. If, however, the heart is diseased, the heart spirit may be disquieted, giving rise to such signs as **vexation**, **susceptibility** to fright, and palpitations, insomnia, or **profuse** dreaming. In serious cases there may be signs either of loss of sensibility such as clouding sleep or **coma**, or of mental disease such as **feeble-mindedness**, **delirious raving**, or **manic** agitation. Therefore, health of the heart and blood directly affects the functions of mental activities (including emotions), consciousness, memory, thinking and sleep.

6   Emotionally, if the heart is strong, spirit will be high; if the heart is weak, spirit will be low. Heart health also determines one's capacity to maintain meaningful relationships—able to give positive energy to others.

7   If heart qi is in excess, a person may show signs of manic depression. Of course, other organ functioning should be considered as influential in any situation.

8   Essence and qi are the physical basis of spirit. If these are strong and flowing smoothly, spirit will be strong. This is why the state of spirit can be observed through the glow of the eyes. Essence, qi and spirit are considered the "three treasures" of the body.

9   Spirit is a transformation of essence and qi. *Ling Shu* (*Spiritual Pivot*[1]) says: "Life comes about through the essence; when the two essences unite, they form the spirit."

Heart qi, heart blood, heart yin and heart yang

10   Heart qi and heart blood form part of the blood and qi of the whole body and represent the basis for the physiologic activity of the heart. When heart qi and heart blood are abundant, the heartbeat is regular, the pulse is moderate and forceful, and the complexion is healthy and **lustrous**. Insufficiency of heart qi and **depletion** of heart blood are characterized by a **lusterless** complexion, **palpitations**, and slow, rapid, or interrupted pulses. Insufficiency of heart qi may lead to blood **stagnation** marked by a green-blue or purple facial complexion and lack of warmth in the extremities. Heart blood depletion leads to impairment of the blood's nourishing function. It may also deprive heart qi of support, giving rise to dizziness, **lassitude** of spirit, shortness of breath, and **copious perspiration**. Heart blood and heart qi are very much interdependent.

11   Heart yin and heart yang refer to the **antagonistic** and **complementary** aspects of the heart's functions. Heart yang refers to a strong heartbeat, smooth blood flow, and the lively, expansive aspect of mental activity. Heart yin refers to a regular, moderate heartbeat and the calm, passive aspect of mental activity. Yin and yang complement and counterbalance each other, ensuring that the heart beats forcefully and regularly, and performs all its normal functions. An essential **prerequisite** of **mutual** counterbalancing and **coordination** of heart yin and heart yang is an abundance of heart blood and **exuberance** of heart qi. Insufficiency of heart blood or heart qi may lead to **debilitation** of heart yin or heart yang. Since "when yang is deficient there is cold," and "when yin is deficient there is heat," such cases present with signs not only of qi or blood deficiency, but also of deficiency cold or deficiency heat.

Opening into the tongue

12   "The heart opens into the tongue" is identical in meaning to "the tongue is the **sprout** of the heart". These statements imply that disturbances of the heart are invariably reflected in the tongue. The heart is related specifically to the tip of the tongue, but it also influences the color, form and appearance of it. The sense of taste is controlled by the heart. Therefore, disease of the heart can be easily recognized on the tongue. If there is

---

① *Ling Shu* (*Spiritual Pivot*):《灵枢》，又译为：*Miraculous Pivot*。

heat, the tongue will be red, possibly dry with a redder tip. If the heat is severe, ulcers can show on the tongue, and they will be painful. If the heart is weak and blood is deficient, the tongue will be pale and thin. In cases of stagnation of the heart blood, a purple tongue can be observed with dark blood stasis speckles.

13 Speech is also directly affected by the heart (i.e., **stutters**, **aphasia**). If heart qi is in excess, there may also be excessive/inappropriate laughter, over-joy, and non-stop talking.

Controlling sweat

14 Sweat comes from the space between the skin and muscles. Blood and body fluids have a common origin. They **intricately** are a part of one another. Deficiencies in heart qi can cause **spontaneous** sweating; deficiencies in heart yin can cause night sweating. Too much sweat can cause deficiency of body fluids and lead to deficiency of blood.

Reference: WISEMAN N, ELLIS A. The fundamentals of chinese medicine [M]. Brookline, Massachusetts: Paradigm Publications, 1996: 53-54.

New Words

subordinate /sə'bɔːdɪnət/	*a.*	lower in rank or position 下级的,附属的
assimilate /ə'sɪmɪleɪt/	*vt.*	absorb and digest 吸收,消化
nourishment /'nʌrɪʃm(ə)nt/	*n.*	the food necessary for growth, health, and good condition 食物,营养物
extremity /ɪk'stremɪti/	*n.*	the hands and feet 肢体
consciousness /'kɔnʃəsnɪs/	*n.*	the state of being aware of and responsive to one's surroundings 意识
vexation /vek'seɪʃ(ə)n/	*n.*	the state of being annoyed, frustrated, or worried 心烦,忧虑,恼怒
susceptibility /sə,septɪ'bɪlɪti/	*n.*	the state or act of being likely or liable to be influenced or harmed by a particular thing 易受影响或损害的状态
profuse /prə'fjuːs/	*a.*	very plentiful, abundant 丰富的,大量的
coma /'kəumə/	*n.*	a prolonged state of deep unconsciousness 昏迷
feeble-mindedness /ˌfiːb(ə)l 'maɪndɪdnəs/	*n.*	having less than average intelligence 低能,愚痴
delirious /dɪ'lɪrɪəs/	*a.*	in an acutely disturbed state of mind characterized by restlessness, illusion, and incoherence 精神错乱的,发狂的
rave /reɪv/	*vi.*	talk incoherently, as if one were delirious or mad 胡言乱语,咆哮
manic /'mænɪk/	*a.*	relating to or affected by mania 躁狂的, 患躁狂病的

笔记

lustrous /ˈlʌstrəs/	a.	having luster, shining 光亮的,有光泽的
depletion /dɪˈpliːʃn/	n.	reduction in the number or quantity of something 消耗,用尽,耗减
lusterless /ˈlʌstələs/	a.	not bright or shiny 没有光泽的
palpitation /ˌpælpɪˈteɪʃ(ə)n/	n.	a noticeably rapid, strong, or irregular heartbeat due to agitation, exertion, or illness 心悸
stagnation /stægˈneɪʃ(ə)n/	n.	the state of not flowing or moving 淤塞,停滞
lassitude /ˈlæsɪtjuːd/	n.	a state of physical or mental weariness; lack of energy 懒怠
copious /ˈkəʊpɪəs/	a.	abundant in supply or quantity 丰富的,大量的
perspiration /ˌpɜːspɪˈreɪʃ(ə)n/	n.	the process of sweating 出汗,流汗
antagonistic /ænˌtæg(ə)ˈnɪstɪk/	a.	active opposition of hostility towards someone or sth. 敌对的,反对的
complementary /ˌkɔmplɪˈment(ə)ri/	a.	combing in such a way as to enhance or emphasize the qualities of each other or another 互补的,补充的
prerequisite /priːˈrekwɪzɪt/	n.	a prior condition for sth. else to happen or exist 先决条件
mutual /ˈmjuːtʃ(ə)l/	a.	a feeling or action experienced or done by each of two or more parties towards the other or others 相互的,共有的
coordination /kəʊˌɔːdɪˈneɪʃ(ə)n/	n.	the organization of the different elements of a complex body or activity so as to enable them to work together effectively 协调,和谐
exuberance /egˈz(j)uːb(ə)r(ə)ns/	n.	the quality of being full of energy, excitement, and cheerfulness 丰富,充沛,充盈
debilitation /dɪˌbɪlɪˈteɪʃ(ə)n/	n.	weakening and loss of energy 虚弱,无力,乏力
sprout /spraʊt/	n.	a shoot of a plant 发芽
stutter /ˈstʌtə/	n.	a tendency to talk with continued involuntary repetition of sounds 结巴
aphasia /əˈfeɪzɪə/	n.	inability to understand or produce speech 失语

笔记

| intricately /'ɪntrɪkətli/ | *ad.* | in a very complicated or detailed manner 盘根错节地 |
| spontaneous /spɒn'teɪnɪəs/ | *a* | (of a process or event) occurring without apparent external cause 自发的 |

Phrases and expressions

govern blood and vessels	主血脉
essence of grain and water	水谷精微
supply of blood	供血
store the spirit	藏神
mental faculty	智力,智能
give rise to	引起
susceptibility to fright	易惊
be in excess	过盛
interrupted pulse	结代脉
blood stagnation	血滞
heart blood depletion	心血耗竭
lassitude of spirit	神疲
shortness of breath	气短
copious perspiration	多汗
sprout of the heart	心之苗
body fluid	津液
spontaneous sweating	自汗
night sweating	盗汗

Task One　Preview

1. Learn the following roots and affixes. Write out the Chinese meaning of the given words.

Roots/ affixes	Meaning of roots/affixes	Words	Chinese meaning of the given words
a-	no or without	amenorrhea	_____
		aphasia	_____
-istic	of or pertaining to	antagonistic	_____
		humanistic	_____
-less	without	lusterless	_____
		restless	_____

my (o)	muscle	myocardial	_____
		myocarditis	_____
non-	not	nontrivial	_____
		nonverbal	_____
-opsy	view of	autopsy	_____
		biopsy	_____
pha/phe	say, speak	aphasia	_____
		prophecy	_____
pre-	before	premature	_____
		prerequisite	_____
pro-	many	profuse	_____
		prolific	_____
re-	again	reabsorption	_____
		redefine	_____
ren (o)	kidney	renal	_____
		renin	_____
simil	alike/same	assimilate	_____
		similar	_____
-scopy	examination	colonoscopy	_____
		gastroscopy	_____
-some	body	chromosome	_____
		ribosome	_____
sub-	under	subcostal	_____
		subcutaneous	_____
ultra-	super	ultrasound	_____
		ultraviolet	_____
ur (o)	urine	uremia	_____
		urology	_____
vas (o)	vessel	vascular	_____
		vasospasm	_____

2. Write down the questions you would like to ask or discuss about the text.

_____

_____

_____

Task Two　Vocabulary

Choose the word or phrase that can best complete the statements.

1) Medicine is _____ to human survival.

48

  A. grateful   B. essential   C. potential   D. potent

2) Like the continuing advance of theories in social science and natural science, TCM theory has to keep _____ with times.

  A. beat   B. path   C. pace   D. neck

3) The devastating pandemic diseases that occurred in European history _____ the lives of tens of millions of people.

  A. exclaimed   B. claimed   C. proclaimed   D. reclaimed

4) Thanks to a great effort in sorting out and organizing classical works during the Qing Dynasty, many TCM classics have been well _____.

  A. deserved   B. served   C. reserved   D. preserved

5) The _____ view of yin-yang theory is considered to be dialectical materialism.

  A. holistic   B. reductive   C. individual   D. practical

6) Variolation (人痘接种) was developed in the 16th century in China as a method to _____ people against smallpox.

  A. subject   B. inherit   C. encompass   D. immunize

7) As to the etiology of brain abscess (脓肿), there have been _____ changes in the last 20 years.

  A. considerate   B. considerable   C. considering   D. inconsiderate

8) The main reason for adverse effects is contamination and inappropriate use rather than _____ risks with herbs themselves.

  A. interior   B. inside   C. inherent   D. inactive

9) It may be true that Chinese medicine's proven ability to absorb ideas and influences will benefit its therapeutic competence in the _____ world.

  A. contemporary   B. competitive   C. temporary   D. epidemic

10) Chinese medicine is built on the traditional Chinese _____, which regards humanities and natural sciences as an integration.

  A. custom   B. pathology   C. physiology   D. philosophy

11) Artemisinin (青蒿素) showed a promising degree of inhibition against _____ growth.

  A. virus   B. parasite   C. bacterium   D. insect

12) The _____ of Artemisinin at a low temperature might be necessary to preserve antimalarial activity.

  A. excerption   B. exploitation   C. extraction   D. exploration

13) In the UK, many patients _____ complementary medicine themselves, and in doing so are trying to develop their own integrated care pathway to improve health outcomes.

  A. access   B. enter   C. contact   D. apply

14) Electro-acupuncture involves a process of electrical stimulation of acupuncture points. An electrical _____ is transmitted through wires attached to acupunctoscope.

  A. conduction   B. impulse   C. pulse   D. pulsation

笔记

15) Cupping is a method of treating disease by causing local _____.

    A. accumulation   B. aggregation   C. congestion   D. infarction

Task Three   Translation

Translate the following expressions into English.

1) 五脏   2) 六腑

3) 滑脉   4) 涩脉

5) 升降出入   6) 浊阴

7) 二阴   8) 阴阳失调

9) 正气   10) 实热证

11) 虚寒证   12) 补虚泻实

13) 辛甘之品   14) 温补阳气

15) 主血脉   16) 四肢厥冷

17) 气短   18) 心悸失眠

19) 气血津液   20) 心开窍于舌

PART III   TRANSLATION AND WRITING

How to Define a Term

In a written definition, we need to make clear in a complete and formal way our understanding of a term. Such a definition usually starts with one meaning of a term. The meaning is then illustrated with a series of details such as facts, examples, or anecdotes that readers will understand.

There are several ways to define a term. 1) Define by function（从功能定义）: Explain what something does or how something works; 2) Define by structure（从结构定义）: Tell how something is organized or put together; 3) Define by analysis（通过分析定义）: Compare the term to other members of its class and then illustrate the differences. These differences are special characteristics that make the term stand out.

The following are definitions of various terms commonly used in Chinese medicine.

1) Upbearing and effusion is the upward and outward movement of qi, a function governed by the liver.

升发是肝的功能，指气向上向外的运动。

2) Defensive qi is yang qi that moves outside the vessels, protecting the body surface and warding off external pathogens.

卫气是人体阳气，行于脉外，具有保卫肌表、抗御外邪的作用。

3) Essential qi theory is one of the basic theories in TCM about qi, the essential part of which constitutes the body and maintains the activities of life, visceral function and metabolism.

精气学说是中医关于气的基本理论之一，精气是构成人体和维持生命活动、脏腑功能和代谢功能的基本物质。

4) Spleen yin is the yin fluid of the spleen, in opposition to spleen yang, referring to the moistening, nourishing and astringing aspect of the spleen.

脾阴是存在于脾脏的阴液，与脾阳相对，指脾脏濡润、滋养和收敛的属性。

5) Kidneys are a pair of organs located in the lumbar region, which store vital essence, promote growth, development, reproduction, and urinary function, and also have a direct effect on the condition of the bone and marrow, activities of the brain, hearing and inspiratory function of the respiratory system.

肾是一对位于腰部的器官，主藏精，主生长、发育、生殖，主水。肾也对骨、髓和脑有直接影响，主听力，主纳气。

6) The heart is located in the thoracic cavity between the two lobes of the lung, above the diaphragm and enveloped by pericardium externally.

心脏位于胸腔内，两肺之间，膈肌之上，裹以心包。

7) Blood is the red fluid circulating through the blood vessels, and nourishing and moistening the whole body. Blood is mainly composed of the nutrient qi and body fluid. It is red in color and sticky in texture. It is vital to the maintenance of life.

51

血液是循行于脉管内濡养全身的红色液态物质,由营气和津液构成,色红质黏,是维持人体生命活动的重要物质。

8) *Sanjiao* (Triple-energizer) is a collective term for the three portions of the body cavity, through which the visceral qi is transformed.

三焦为人体上、中、下焦的合称,是脏腑之气转化的通道。

9) Static blood is a pathological product of blood stagnation, including extravasated blood and the blood circulating sluggishly or blood congested in a viscus, all of which may turn into pathogenic factor.

瘀血是血滞的病理产物,凡溢于脉外的血液或血液运行不畅而停滞于脏器之中的部分都叫瘀血,可转化为病理因素。

10) Kidney deficiency is a general term for deficiency conditions of the kidney, including kidney yin deficiency, kidney yang deficiency, insufficiency of kidney essence, and insecurity of kidney qi.

肾虚一般指肾阴虚、肾阳虚、肾精不足、肾气不固等各种肾虚证的总称。

11) Heat scorching kidney yin refers to the damage to kidney yin by pathogenic heat, usually occurring in the advanced stage of warm heat disease.

热灼肾阴指温热病后期肾阴被热邪所消耗。

12) Delicate viscus is an expression referring to the lung which is the viscus most susceptible to invasion by external pathogens.

娇脏指肺脏,指肺容易感受外邪。

13) Thoracic accumulation is a diseased state attributable to accumulation of pathogens, such as heat or cold in combination with retained fluid or phlegm or stagnant food, in the chest and abdomen, often manifested by local rigidity, fullness and tenderness.

结胸证是胸腹中原有水饮、痰或积食与热或寒邪互结而成的病证,常表现为(颈项)强硬、(胸腹)胀满、局部有触痛。

14) Heat entering the blood level is a pathological change characterized by the pathogenic heat entering the blood aspect, causing hemorrhages, mental disturbances, and even convulsions.

热入血分指以邪热侵入血分为特点的病变,表现为出血、躁扰不安,甚或抽搐。

15) Qi transformation is a general term referring to various changes through the activity of qi, namely the metabolism and mutual transformation between essence, qi, blood and body fluids.

气化是指通过气的运动而产生的各种变化的概称,具体指精、气、血、津液的新陈代谢及其相互转化。

Sample

Holistic Medicine

1) Holistic medicine is a term used to describe therapies that attempt to treat the patient as a whole person. Instead of treating an illness, as in orthodox allopathy (对抗疗法), holistic medicine looks at an individual's overall physical, mental, spiritual and emotional

wellbeing before recommending treatment. 2) A practitioner with a holistic approach treats the symptoms of illness as well as looking for the underlying cause of the illness. Holistic medicine also attempts to prevent illness by placing a greater emphasis on optimizing health. The body's systems are regarded as interdependent parts of the person's whole being. Its natural state is one of health, and an illness or disease is an imbalance in the body's systems. 3) Holistic therapies tend to emphasize proper nutrition and avoidance of substances—such as chemicals—that pollute the body. Their techniques are non-invasive.

Some of the world's health systems that are holistic in nature include naturopathic medicine, homeopathy, and TCM. Many alternative or natural therapies, although not always the case, have a holistic approach. 4) The term complementary medicine is used to refer to the use of both allopathic and holistic treatments. It is more often used in Great Britain, but is gaining acceptance in the United States.

There are no limits to the range of diseases and disorders that can be treated in a holistic way, as 5) the principle of holistic healing is to balance the body, mind, spirit and emotions so that the person's whole being functions smoothly. When an individual seeks holistic treatment for a particular illness or condition, other health problems are relieved without direct treatment, due to improvement in the performance of the immune system, which is one of the goals of holistic medicine.

Task One　Translation

Translate the underlined parts in the above sample into Chinese.

1) _____

_____

2) _____

_____

3) _____

_____

4) _____

_____

5) _____

_____

Task Two　Writing

Choose a term of Chinese medicine and write a 200-word composition about it, incorporating its definition. Try to use as many sentence patterns as possible in PART Ⅲ. Alternatively, you may work in pairs on a chosen term, search the information on the internet, write the definition and then present it to the class.

_____

_____

_____

PART IV　REFLECTION

Traditional Chinese medicine (TCM) uses terminology that is difficult for other cultures rooted in modern science to understand. In 2007, WHO published a dictionary-type book entitled *WHO International Standard Terminologies on Traditional Medicine in the Western Pacific Regions* which has a total of 3,543 technical terms that are commonly used in traditional Chinese (TCM), Japanese (Kampo), Korean (TKM) and Vietnamese (TVM) medicines. In this comprehensive guide, each term has the English expression, the original Chinese character and a concise English definition. It is a milestone in codifying the wisdom of TCM. In 2022, WHO issued *WHO International Standard Terminologies on Traditional Chinese Medicine*. It includes a total of 3,415 terms, among which 3,387 terms have detailed descriptions and 28 are terms of main categorization.

Read the books and search the internet for more information on **the translation of TCM terminology** and think about the following questions:

1) How are you going to make use of the books?

2) Have you found any problems with some translations? If yes, how would you improve those translations?

Unit 3

Diagnosis and Therapeutic Principles of Traditional Chinese Medicine

LEARNING OUTCOMES

This unit offers you opportunities to:
- **collect** the signs and symptoms by using the four examinations
- **use** the terms related to diagnosis and therapeutic principles of traditional Chinese medicine (TCM)
- **describe/introduce** a pattern of TCM
- **compare** a pattern to another similar pattern
- **reflect on** the importance of pattern differentiation

笔记

PART I   LISTENING AND SPEAKING

Before you listen

In this section you will hear a short passage entitled "Four Methods of Traditional Chinese Medicine". The following words and phrases may be of help.

restore /rɪ'stɔː/	vt.	使恢复,修复
reflect /rɪ'flekt/	vt.	表达,显示
detective /dɪ'tektɪv/	n.	侦探
clue /kluː/	n.	线索
four methods of diagnosis		四诊

While you listen

Listen to the passage carefully and fill in each of the blanks marked from 1) to 10) according to what you have heard.

ER-3-1
Listening
practice

Four Methods of Traditional Chinese Medicine

In traditional Chinese medicine (TCM), there are four methods of diagnosis. The first method is looking or inspection. The physician may 1)_____ your eyes, your face, your skin and examine your tongue because it 2)_____ your health. The second method is asking questions or inquiry, such as "Do you 3)_____ cold drinks or hot ones?"

The third method is auscultation and olfaction, or 4)_____, a very small part but still important of a diagnosis. Auscultation refers to listening to a patient's voice, speech, 5)_____, coughing and so on. Olfaction refers to detecting the 6)_____ of a patient's body, secretions, excretions and so on by smelling. The fourth method is 7)_____ and palpation. Pulse examination is also called pulse-taking, meaning a physician uses his finger to feel and press a patient's pulse to know the 8)_____ of his or her health. Palpation means a physician touches or presses a certain part of the patient's body. The doctors are really like a detective. They put all the clues together to 9)_____ and develop a treatment program to 10)_____ for the patient.

After you listen

Please discuss with your partner the following questions and give your presentation to the class.

1) How can a TCM practitioner make a correct diagnosis?
2) Why is a TCM practitioner like a detective?

PART II　READING

Text A

Principles and Strategies of Treatment

1　Most conditions we see in practice are characterized by multiple patterns and a **coexistence** of deficiency and excess. Thus, although our diagnosis of the patterns involved may be absolutely correct, the success of the treatment depends very much on the adoption of the correct strategy and method of treatment. For example, although we may correctly diagnose a condition as spleen deficiency and dampness, should we concentrate on **tonifying** the former, **eliminating** the latter or doing both simultaneously? In my experience, the adoption of the correct treatment principle in deciding whether to tonify the body's qi or eliminate pathogenic factors is absolutely **crucial** to the success of the treatment.

2　One point of view from which the principles of treatment are discussed is about the "root" and the "manifestation". The root is called "*ben*" in Chinese, which literally means "root", and the manifestation is called "*biao*", which literally means "outward sign" or "manifestation", i.e., the outward manifestation of some inner, unseen root. The root and manifestation can be compared to a tree, its root being the root and its branches the manifestation.

3　When considering the root and manifestation, it is important to understand the connection between the two. They are not separate entities, but two aspects of a contradiction, like yin and yang. As their names suggest, they are related to one another, just as the roots of a tree are connected to its branches, the former under the ground and invisible, the latter above the ground and visible. The same relationship exists between the root of a disease and its clinical manifestations: They are **indissolubly** related and they form two aspects of the same entity. There is no separation between the two. The art of diagnosis consists precisely in identifying the root (i.e., the root of symptoms and signs) by looking at the manifestation (i.e., the clinical manifestations).

4　Generally speaking, the root is primary and is treated first. However, under certain circumstances, the manifestation can become primary and needs to be treated first, even though the **ultimate** aim is always to treat the root. The decision to treat the root or the manifestation depends on the severity and **urgency** of the clinical manifestations. There are three possible courses of action: 1) Treat the root only; 2) Treat both the root and the manifestation; 3) Treat the manifestation first, and the root later.

Treat the root only

5　Generally speaking, treating the root only is sufficient to clear all clinical manifestations in most cases. The method of treating the root can be used in **interior** or **exterior** as well as chronic or **acute** diseases. The approach of treating the root only is **applicable** in cases

57

when the clinical manifestations are not too **severe**. If the clinical manifestations are severe or even life threatening, the approach should be changed, as will be explained below.

Treat both the root and the manifestation

6   This approach is widely used in practice. In chronic cases when the clinical manifestations are severe and **distressing** for the patient, it is necessary to treat both the root and the manifestation simultaneously. This approach is also applied when the clinical manifestations themselves are such that they would **perpetuate** the original problem. For example, in the case of a woman with qi deficiency leading to excessive **menstrual** bleeding[①] (qi not holding blood), **prolonged** menstrual bleeding over many years will in itself lead to further deficiency of both qi and blood.

7   In the case of a patient suffering from spleen-yang deficiency causing severe **edema**, the correct approach would again be to treat both the root (i.e., tonify and warm the spleen) and the manifestation (i.e., eliminate edema).

8   In the case of a child who has severe **whooping** cough caused by **phlegm**-heat in the lung, it would be necessary again to adopt the method of treating both the root (by clearing lung-heat and resolving phlegm) and the manifestation (by stopping the cough). This is the correct approach since the coughing is very distressing and debilitating to the child, so it would be wrong to simply treat the root and wait for the symptoms to improve. This example can be compared and contrasted with a case of a chronic slight dry cough caused by yin deficiency, in which case the cough is not bad or serious enough to **warrant** treating the manifestation.

Treat the manifestation first and the root later

9   Under certain circumstances the root becomes secondary and the manifestation needs to be treated first, and usually urgently too. This approach is applicable in all cases when the clinical manifestations are very severe or even life-threatening: this is especially common in acute cases.

10   For example, a patient has a **productive** cough with profuse watery phlegm, **breathlessness**, chilliness, a thick sticky tongue coating and a slippery pulse. The clinical manifestations reflect spleen-yang deficiency (the root) causing **retention** of phlegm in the lungs (the manifestation). In this case, if the clinical manifestations are severe and acute (particularly in an elderly person), the correct approach is to deal with the manifestation first, by resolving phlegm and stimulating the **descending** of lung-qi.[②] Later, when the symptoms of phlegm have **subsided**, one can treat the root (i.e., tonify and warm the spleen).

11   Another example is a woman suffering from **dysmenorrhea** caused by stasis of blood due to deficiency of qi. In this case, the correct approach is to concentrate on treating the manifestation (i.e., move blood and stop pain) before or during the **period**, and treating the

---

① excessive menstrual bleeding: 月经过多。西医专业用语是 menorrhagia。

② resolving phlegm and stimulating the descending of lung-qi: 可理解为 "降气化痰"。

笔记

root (i.e., tonify qi) just after and in between periods.

12　It should be noted that, although in many cases the root **coincides** with a deficiency and the manifestation with a pathogenic factor,[①] this is by no means always so. The case of a spleen-qi deficiency (root) leading to dampness (manifestations) and that of liver-blood deficiency (root) leading to liver-yang rising (manifestations) are common examples in which the root is a deficient pattern and the manifestation an excess one.

13　However, there are many cases when this is not so. An exterior **invasion** of a pathogenic factor is an obvious example in which the root (e.g. external wind) is an excess condition. In the case of cold **congealing** in the **uterus** and causing blood stasis, both the root (cold) and the manifestation (blood stasis) are excess conditions. Finally, an excess-type manifestation can itself become a root. Phlegm is a common example of this as phlegm itself is an excess-type manifestation deriving from a deficient root (spleen and kidney deficiency). After a prolonged time, phlegm itself can become a cause of further pathology and therefore turn into a root.

Reference: MACIOCIA G. The foundations of Chinese medicine [M]. 3rd ed. New York: Churchill Livingstone, 2015:1171-1180.

New words

strategy /ˈstrætɪdʒi/	n.	a plan of action designed to achieve a long-term or overall aim 策略
coexistence /ˌkəʊɪgˈzɪstəns/	n.	the state or fact of living or existing at the same time or in the same place 共存
tonify /ˈtəʊnɪfaɪ/	vt.	(of acupuncture or herbal medicine) increase the available energy of (a bodily part or system) 补养,补益
eliminate /ɪˈlɪmɪneɪt/	vt.	expel (waste matter) from the body 消除
crucial /ˈkruːʃ(ə)l/	a.	of great importance 关键性的
indissolubly /ˌɪndɪˈsɒljʊbli/	ad.	in a way that is unable to be destroyed, undone, or broken 不可分解地
ultimate /ˈʌltɪmət/	a.	being or happening at the end of a process; final 最后的
urgency /ˈəːdʒ(ə)nsi/	n.	importance requiring swift action 紧急
interior /ɪnˈtɪərɪə/	a.	situated on or relating to the inside of sth. 内部的
exterior /ɪkˈstɪərɪə/	a.	forming, situated on, or relating to the outside of sth. 外部的
acute /əˈkjuːt/	a.	(of a disease or its symptoms) severe but of short duration 急性的

---

① root coincides with a deficiency and the manifestation with a pathogenic factor: 可理解为"本虚标实"。

applicable /əˈplɪkəb(ə)l/	a.	relevant or appropriate 适当的
severe /sɪˈvɪə/	a.	(of sth. bad or undesirable) very great 严重的
distress /dɪˈstres/	vt.	cause (someone) anxiety, sorrow, or pain 使痛苦
perpetuate /pəˈpetʃʊeɪt/	vt.	make (sth.) continue indefinitely 保持
menstrual /ˈmenstrʊəl/	a.	relating to the menses or menstruation 月经的
prolonged /prəˈlɒŋd/	a.	continuing for a long time or longer than usual 延长的
edema /ɪˈdiːmə/	n.	a condition characterized by an excess of watery fluid collecting in the cavities or tissues of the body 水肿
whoop /wuːp/	vi.	make the paroxysmal (阵发性) gasp characteristic of whooping cough 喘息
phlegm /flem/	n.	the thick viscous substance secreted by the mucous membranes of the respiratory passages, especially when produced in excessive quantities during a cold 痰
warrant /ˈwɔr(ə)nt/	vt.	justify or necessitate (a course of action) 保证
productive /prəˈdʌktɪv/	a.	(of a cough) that raises mucus from the respiratory tract 多产的
breathlessness /ˈbreθləsnəs/	n.	gasping for breath, typically due to exertion 喘不过气
retention /rɪˈtenʃ(ə)n/	n.	failure to eliminate a substance from the body 滞留
descend /dɪˈsend/	vi.	move or fall downwards 下降
subside /səbˈsaɪd/	vi.	become less intense, violent, or severe 减弱
dysmenorrhea /ˌdɪsmenəˈriːə/	n.	painful menstruation, typically involving abdominal cramps 痛经
period /ˈpɪərɪəd/	n.	(also menstrual period) a flow of blood and other material from the lining of the uterus, lasting for a few days and occurring in sexually mature women who are not pregnant at intervals of about one lunar month until the menopause 月经

笔记

60

coincide /ˌkəʊɪn'saɪd/	vi.	occur at the same time 同时发生
invasion /ɪn'veɪʒ(ə)n/	n.	an incursion（侵入）by a large number of people or things into a place or sphere of activity 侵袭
congeal /kən'dʒiːl/	vi.	become semi-solid, especially on cooling 凝结
uterus /'juːt(ə)rəs/	n.	(pl. uteri or uteruses) the organ in the lower body of a woman or female mammal where offspring are conceived and in which they gestate（孕育）before birth 子宫

Phrases and expressions

coexistence of deficiency and excess	虚实夹杂
spleen deficiency and dampness	脾虚夹湿
separate entity	独立体
two aspects of a contradiction	矛盾的两个方面
qi not holding blood	气不摄血
deficiency of both qi and blood	气血两虚
eliminate edema	消肿
whooping cough	百日咳
clearing lung-heat and resolving phlegm	清肺化痰
stop the cough	止咳
dry cough	干咳
tongue coating	舌苔
slippery pulse	脉滑
retention of phlegm in the lung	痰浊阻肺
stasis of blood	血瘀
move blood and stop pain	行血止痛
during the period	月经期间
coincide with	同时发生
exterior invasion of a pathogenic factor	外感病邪
cold congealing in the uterus	寒凝胞宫
a cause of further pathology	继发性病理因素

Task One   Preview

1. Learn the following word roots and affixes. Write out the Chinese meaning of the given words.

Roots/ Affixes	Meaning of roots/affixes	Words	Chinese meaning of the given words
ab-	go bad	abnormality	_____
		abuse	_____
co-	together	coexistence	_____
		coincide	_____
contra-	opposite	contradiction	_____
		contravention	_____
de-	reduce	debilitating	_____
		descending	_____
dia-	through	diagnosis	_____
		dialectic	_____
dys-	bad	dysmenorrhea	_____
		dyspepsia	_____
hyper-	excessive	hypersensitivity	_____
		hypertension	_____
hyster (o)	uterus	hysterectomy	_____
		hysteromyoma	_____
inter-	inward	interior	_____
		internal	_____
labi (o)	lip	labiodental	_____
		labioplasty	_____
men (o)	menstruation	menopause	_____
		menostasis	_____
mid-	middle	midposition	_____
		midsection	_____
multi-	many	multimedia	_____
		multiple	_____
-ness	the state or quality of	dizziness	_____
		heaviness	_____
-pathy	disease	cardiopathy	_____
		rhinopathy	_____
scend	climb	ascend	_____
		descend	_____

solu/solv	loosen	dissolve	_____
		indissolubly	_____
uter	uterus	uterine	_____
		uterus	_____

2. Write down the questions you would like to ask or discuss about the text.

_____

_____

_____

Task Two   Speaking

1. Answer the following questions according to the text.

1) What does the success of a treatment depend on?

2) What is the relationship between the root and the manifestation?

3) What does the decision to treat the root or the manifestation depend on?

4) In what cases should the approach of treating the root only be used?

5) How should a doctor treat the patient suffering from spleen-yang deficiency causing severe edema?

6) How should a child be treated if he/she has severe whooping cough caused by phlegm-heat in the lung?

7) In what cases should the approach of treating the manifestation first and the root later be adopted?

8) When is it necessary to treat both the root and the manifestation simultaneously?

2. Work in pairs or groups and exchange views on the following case study.

A Case Study of Migraine Headache

In October 2011, a 32-year-old Ethiopian-American woman, height and weight proportionate, presented with a 10-year history of debilitating migraine headaches. She described them as the worst feeling of her life, with a pain scale rating of 10 out of 10 (10 being the highest level of pain). During the attacks, the patient experienced sharp pain, photophobia (畏光), distorted vision with visible auras, a feeling of heaviness, dizziness, and irritability, occasional nausea and vomiting, hypersensitivity to sound, and a desire to lie down in a dark, noise-free room. The pain was often on the right side of her head, occurring once every 7 to 10 days.

MRI and computed tomography (CT) scans were taken 2 years before by a neurologist and showed no abnormalities. The patient reported no previous major illnesses or surgeries, no family history of illness, and no use of medications or nutritional supplements.

The TCM intake revealed that the patient had cold hands and feet with a warm midsection. She sweated easily and craved chocolate, ice cream, and fried foods. She suffered from sinus congestion (鼻窦充血) and allergies. She vomited and felt nauseated weekly. Once or twice a week, she was constipated with occasional blood in the bowel due to excessive strain to clear bowels. She was prone to stress and anxiety. The patient had an intrauterine device（宫内节育器, IUD）, and her last menstrual cycle was May 2010. The patient had a slightly red, swollen, and scalloped tongue（齿痕舌）with a thin yellow coating. The sublingual veins（舌下静脉）were dark and full. The right pulse was slippery. The left pulse was slippery with a wiry and stronger *guan* position than the right *guan* position.

Reference: PAYANT M J. A single case study: treating migraine headache with acupuncture, chinese herbs, and diet [J/OL]. Global advances in health and medicine, 2014, 3 (1):71-74. [2022-09-22]. http://www.ncbi.nlm.nih.gov/pmc/articles/PMC3921614/. DOI: 10.7453/gahmj.2013.060.

Topic for discussion: Please give the following information according to the above case study: 1) general information (age, gender, and ethnicity); 2) main complaints; 3) history of present illness (signs, symptoms, tongue, and pulse condition); 4) past medical history; and 5) family history.

Task Three   Vocabulary

1. Match up each word in Column A with its appropriate definition from Column B.

Column A	Column B
1) pattern	a. cause (someone) anxiety, sorrow, or pain
2) tonify	b. make (someone) very weak and infirm
3) distress	c. a condition characterized by an excess of watery fluid collecting in the cavities or tissues of the body
4) whoop	d. gasping for breath, typically due to exertion
5) chronic	e. relating to the menses or menstruation
6) edema	f. the thick viscous substance secreted by the mucous membranes of the respiratory passages
7) menstrual	g. (of an illness) persisting for a long time or constantly recurring
	h. a long rasping indrawn breath, characteristic of whooping cough
8) phlegm	
	i. (of acupuncture or herbal medicine) increase the available energy of (a bodily part or system)
9) breathlessness	
	j. a diagnostic concept and a summary of the location, cause, nature, and condition of a disease
10) dysmenorrhea	
	k. painful menstruation, typically involving abdominal cramps
11) uterus	l. the organ in the lower body of a woman or female mammal where offspring are conceived and in which they gestate before birth
12) debilitate	

2. Fill in the blanks with the words given below. Change the form where necessary.

clearance	pattern	reduce	deficient	describe
menopause	tonification	imbalance	excess	pulse
menstruation	palpation	diagnose	prescription	examine

笔记

64

Traditional Chinese Medicine Diagnosis

Diagnosis in traditional Chinese medicine (TCM) may appear to be simply a grouping of symptoms, but the elegance of TCM is that a diagnosis automatically indicates a treatment strategy. For example, a woman experiencing 1) _____ may have hot flashes, night sweats, thirst, and irritability. This group of symptoms is described as kidney yin deficiency with heat. It immediately points to the indicated therapy: 2) _____ kidney yin and 3) _____ deficiency heat. Since standard formulas are available for this pattern, such as Rehmannia Teapills, an accurate diagnosis enables a practitioner to 4) _____ a treatment that has been proved safe and effective for thousands of years.

A practitioner can obtain all of the information needed to diagnose a disease through four examinations which include inspection, auscultation and olfaction (or listening and smelling), inquiry as well as 5) pulse taking and_____. Simply by using these four diagnostic methods, traditional practitioners can accurately assess physical and emotional 6) _____ of the internal organs and reestablish harmony.

In TCM, diagnostic indicators are always viewed holistically. For example, fatigue is a symptom of qi or blood 7) _____, but fatigue is also a symptom in a case of wind cold. If a person with wind cold was mistakenly 8) _____ with qi deficiency, he might be given ginseng, a strong tonic that would make the symptoms much worse.

A careful practitioner would note that the person's 9) _____ was strong and floating, a sign of wind cold; by contrast, a person with qi deficiency would have a deep and weak pulse. While it is necessary to learn the individual diagnostic 10) _____, it is crucial to remember that any sign or symptom must be viewed in relation to the whole person.

Reference: SCHOENBART B, SHEFI E. Traditional Chinese medicine diagnosis [EB/OL]. (2007-08-12) [2015-10-09]. http://health.howstuffworks.com/wellness/natural-medicine/chinese/traditional-chinese-medicine-diagnosis.htm.

Task Four   Translation

1. Study the following sentences and pay attention to the underlined parts.

1) The method of treating the root can be used in interior or exterior as well as chronic or acute diseases. (para. 5)

2) If the clinical manifestations are severe or even life threatening, the approach should be changed. (para. 5)

3) This example can be compared and contrasted with a case of a chronic slight dry cough caused by yin deficiency. (para. 8)

4) The clinical manifestations reflect spleen-yang deficiency causing retention of phlegm in the lungs. (para. 10)

5) Later, when the symptoms of phlegm have subsided, one can treat the root. (para. 10)

6) Another example is a woman suffering from dysmenorrhea caused by stasis of blood due to deficiency of qi. (para. 11)

笔记

2. Translate the following sentences into English.

1) 扶正法可用于治疗虚证。

2) 如果是虚实夹杂证,治疗方法应该调整。

3) 这种病证可与外感风寒导致的急性咳嗽进行比较。

4) 这些症状和体征反映脾气虚导致了痰湿阻滞中焦。

5) 当疾病不再威胁到生命之后,我们可针对"本"进行治疗。

6) 这位患者的水肿是由脾肾阳虚导致的。

Text B

The Four Examinations

1   Traditional Chinese medicine (TCM) rests on what is called the four examinations of diagnosis. They are looking, listening/smelling, asking and palpation.

2   This is **deceptively** simple. In TCM there are many, many systems and microsystems that can be examined and **plundered** for information, and nearly all of them rest on the assumption that the **microcosm** reflects the **macrocosm**. That is, a small area, like the ear or the pulse, is a **holographic** representation of the larger whole of the human body. This means that nearly any part of the body can be an image of the entire body. The methods that I list here are only a few of the major ones.

Looking

3   One thing that almost everyone has at least amateur training in is diagnosis of the face. The simplest way to diagnose from the face is simply to notice the color on a face. However, even this **simplicity** is deceptive, because colors usually do not stand out in **stark** contrast. There are many **subtle** shades that **layer** themselves simultaneously in a face. This means that it requires a lot of visual sensitivity to see that color.

4   Along with color, the luster of the skin is also noted. Things can get much more complicated, though, because every individual feature of the face indicates something about the health of the body. Large ears, for instance, indicate robust kidney qi, and since the kidneys are the root of one's constitutional energy,[①] that means you were born with a lot of energy to spend, so to speak. Every feature correlates with something. The eyebrow area represents the liver/**gall bladder;** the nose represents the lung, etc.

5   Another microsystem is the ear. Some acupuncturists specialize in diagnosing and treating from the ear, and can tell instantly by looking at the ear where someone has pain,

---

① kidneys are the root of one's constitutional energy: 可理解为"肾为先天之本"。

where a woman is in her menstrual cycle, etc. The whole body is often treated through the ear, using needles or seeds. As you can see from the image below, in this case the whole body is represented according to the image of an upside-down **fetus** mapped onto the ear, with the **navel** in the center.

6　One of the most important methods of looking diagnosis is the tongue. Many details of the tongue are examined, including qualities such as color, size, shape, depressions, swollen areas, enlarged **papillae**, **moisture**, thickness and color of coating as well as movement.

Listening/Smelling

7　The voice is classified into roughly five types—shout, laugh, sing, weep, **groan**— according to the five phases system of TCM, which correlates each element with a set of organs; thus, the sounds heard in the voice can be used to determine which organ systems are disordered.

8　Smelling is classified with listening as one of the "four examinations", under a similar set of assumptions. Practically speaking, it is much less commonly used, in part because humans are not very **odor**-centric.

Asking

9　Traditional diagnosis centers around the "Ten Questions". TCM practitioners ask people about a broad variety of things, beginning with the main complaint, but branching out and including tension/pain, energy, sleep, **digestion**, thirst, menstruation, urine, bowel movements, sweating, mental functioning, emotional functioning, relationships, and even the birth history sometimes.

10　And every little area has other related questions involved. Headache is a good example: Questions may be asked about the location of the headache on the head, the quality of the pain (sharp, dull, **throbbing**, etc.), how often it comes on, what time of day, if it is associated with stress or food, and what makes it better or worse.

Palpation

11　There are many ways to diagnose by palpation. The pulse at the **radial artery** is perhaps the most **iconic** of TCM. Historically, there have been many different kinds of pulse diagnosis, but, again, they all rely on the principle of holographic representation— the idea that information throughout the body can be gathered by focusing attention within a small area of the body.

12　The picture on the above **depicts** six positions (three on each side) and two different depths or pressures[①] at which you assess the pulse, the **superficial** and the deep. This is the standard for many pulse diagnostic systems. Classically there are 28 different qualities that can be found on the pulse.

13　To make things more complicated, there are pulses to be found at many other sites throughout the body, such as on the foot and the head. These are rarely used today by the

---

① two different depths or pressures: 两种不同深度或压力 (说明:诊脉大多取浮、中、沉三候)。

Chinese, but they are used by, among others, Japanese meridian therapists.

14　Another form of diagnosis is the palpation of the abdomen. Once again, there are many maps of the **torso**, and also many ways to palpate. Some doctors have learned to palpate the abdomen with rather strong, firm pressure, while others, like the Japanese style of Toyohari,[①] emphasizes feather-light touch with only occasional pressure, and sensitivity to very slight changes in **texture**, temperature, and firmness of the skin.

15　Palpation of the acupuncture meridians is yet another method of diagnosis. This involves knowing all twelve of the main meridians[②] (also called channels) and where they travel, and feeling the skin to sense, once again, changes in tone, texture, and temperature.

Putting it all together

16　Despite the seeming complexity of all of these systems, the real work is in **integrating** all of this information. In real world situations, much of the information will not match. And this is why diagnosis is an art form: Medical practitioners are like Sherlock Holmes,[③] gathering as many clues as possible, trying to notice the small details that everyone else misses, **sifting** through the information to determine what's relevant and what's not. The diagnostician journeys through the microcosms of the body, peer through the many different lenses, trying like hell to **penetrate** the **veil** of a person's being.

17　The best physician sees to the roots of a problem and is able to **pinpoint** exactly where and how to treat a person, whether it is through an acupuncture point, an herbal formula, or a simple conversation.

　　Reference: YEH D D. The four pillars of diagnosis [EB/OL]. [2015-10-18]. http://acupunctureecology. com/articles/four-pillars-of-diagnosis/.

New Words

deceptively /dɪˈseptɪvli/	*ad.*	in a way or to an extent that gives a misleading impression 迷惑地
plunder /ˈplʌndə/	*vt.*	take material (from artistic or academic work) for one's own purposes 取用
microcosm /ˈmaɪkrə(ʊ)kɒz(ə)m/	*n.*	a community, place, or situation regarded as encapsulating in miniature the characteristics of sth. much larger 微观世界
macrocosm /ˈmækrə(ʊ)kɒz(ə)m/	*n.*	the whole of a complex structure, especially the world or the universe, contrasted with a small or representative part of it 宏观世界

---

①　Japanese style of Toyohari: 日式针灸。
②　twelve of the main meridians: 十二正经。
③　Sherlock Holmes: 夏洛克·福尔摩斯, 19 世纪末英国小说家阿瑟·柯南·道尔塑造的一个才华横溢的侦探。

holographic /ˌhɔləˈgræfɪk/	*a.*	produced using holograms 全息的
simplicity /sɪmˈplɪsɪti/	*n.*	the quality or condition of being easy to understand or do 简单
stark /stɑːk/	*a.*	unpleasantly or sharply clear（对比）鲜明的
subtle /ˈsʌt(ə)l/	*a.*	(especially of a change or distinction) so delicate or precise as to be difficult to analyze or describe 不易察觉的；不明显的
layer /ˈleɪə/	*vt.*	arrange in a layer or layers 把……分层堆放
gall /gɔːl/	*n.*	bile 胆汁
bladder /ˈblædə/	*n.*	anything inflated and hollow 囊状物
fetus /ˈfiːtəs/	*n.*	an unborn offspring of a mammal, in particular an unborn human baby more than eight weeks after conception 胎儿
navel /ˈneɪv(ə)l/	*n.*	a rounded, knotty depression in the center of a person's belly caused by the detachment of the umbilical（脐带的）cord after birth 脐
papilla /pəˈpɪlə/	*n.*	(*pl.* papillae) a small rounded protuberance（突起）on a part or organ of the body 乳头
moisture /ˈmɔɪstʃə/	*n.*	water or other liquid diffused in a small quantity as vapor, within a solid, or condensed on a surface 水分；潮湿
groan /grəʊn/	*n.*	the action or state of making a deep inarticulate sound in response to pain or despair 呻吟
odor /ˈəʊdə/	*n.*	a distinctive smell, especially an unpleasant one 气味
digestion /daɪˈdʒestʃ(ə)n/	*n.*	a person's capacity to digest food 消化
throb /θrɔb/	*vi.*	feel pain in a series of regular beats 抽痛
radial /ˈreɪdɪəl/	*a.*	relating to the radius 桡骨的
artery /ˈɑːtəri/	*a.*	any of the tubes that carry blood from the heart to other parts of the body 动脉
iconic /aɪˈkɔnɪk/	*a.*	of the nature of an icon 符号的，图标的
depict /dɪˈpɪkt/	*vt.*	portray in words; describe 描述

笔记

superficial /ˌsuːpəˈfɪʃ(ə)l/	*a.*	existing or occurring at or on the surface 表层的
torso /ˈtɔːsəʊ/	*n.*	the trunk of the human body 躯干
texture /ˈtekstʃə/	*n.*	the feel, appearance, or consistency of a surface or a substance 质地
integrate /ˈɪntɪɡreɪt/	*vt.*	combine (one thing) with another to form a whole 使整合
sift /sɪft/	*vi.*	examine sth. thoroughly so as to isolate that which is most important and useful 筛选,遴选
penetrate /ˈpenɪtreɪt/	*vt.*	go into or through (sth.), especially with force or effort 穿透
veil /veɪl/	*n.*	a piece of fine material worn by women to protect or conceal the face 面纱
pinpoint /ˈpɪnpɔɪnt/	*vt.*	find or identify with great accuracy or precision 确定,精准定位

Phrases and expressions

four examinations (of diagnosis)	四诊
diagnosis of the face	面诊
gall bladder	胆囊
specialize in	专门研究
menstrual cycle	月经周期
map... onto	映射到
looking diagnosis	望诊
be classified into	分类为
center around	以……为中心
main complaint	主诉
bowel movement	排便
birth history	生育史
quality of the pain	疼痛性质
radial artery	桡动脉
palpation of the abdomen	按腹
palpation of the acupuncture meridians	按经络
twelve (of the main) meridians	十二正经
like hell	拼命地
herbal formula	方剂

Task One   Preview

1. Learn the following word roots and affixes. Write out the Chinese meaning of the given words.

Roots/ Affixes	Meaning of roots/affixes	Words	Chinese meaning of the given words
cardi (o)	heart	cardiac	_____
		cardinal	_____
chron (o)	time	chronic	_____
		chronology	_____
circ	circle	circular	_____
		circulation	_____
dif-	separate	differ	_____
		differentiation	_____
-dynia	pain	cervicodynia	_____
		gastrodynia	_____
-emia	blood condition	anemia	_____
		leukemia	_____
flu (o)	flow	fluency	_____
		fluid	_____
fore-	before, in front	forearm	_____
		forehead	_____
-gram	record	cardiogram	_____
		radiogram	_____
holo-	entire, complete	holographic	_____
		holonomic	_____
hypo-	below, under	hypotension	_____
		hypodermic	_____
macro-	large	macrocosm	_____
		macrosystem	_____
micro-	small	microcosm	_____
		microsystem	_____
migra	wander	migraine	_____
		migrate	_____
pict	paint	depict	_____
		pictograph	_____

radi (o)	radius	radialis	_____
		transradial	_____
semi-	half, part	semiconscious	_____
		semidigested	_____
trans-	transfer	transit	_____
		transportation	_____

2. Write down the questions you would like to ask or discuss about the text.

_____

_____

_____

Task Two　Vocabulary

Choose the word or phrase that can best complete the statements.

1) According to TCM, the pulse can reveal whether a _____ is of hot or cold nature, whether it is of excess or deficiency type.

　　A. pattern　　　　　B. symptom　　　　　C. disease　　　　D. manifestation

2) As the process of disease is complex, the abnormal pulses do not often appear in their pure form; the _____ of two pulses or more is often present.

　　A. integration　　　B. coexistence　　　　C. combination　　　D. unit

3) A bright (shiny), white face can _____ deficiency of qi or a cold condition, while a dull, pale face with no shine is a sign of blood deficiency.

　　A. explain　　　　　B. uncover　　　　　C. express　　　　D. indicate

4) Another important aspect of diagnosis through observation of the tongue is the appearance of the _____ on the tongue.

　　A. quilt　　　　　　B. paint　　　　　　C. layer　　　　　D. coating

5) Someone _____ with yang deficiency may look pale or anemic, have dark circles under their eyes, and will have a weak voice.

　　A. affecting　　　　B. suffering　　　　　C. affected　　　　D. effecting

6) TCM has long been used to treat diabetes in China and many other countries thanks to its safety and _____.

　　A. effectiveness　　B. effect　　　　　　C. efficacy　　　　D. effective

7) Therapeutic _____ should be further selected and determined, including oral use of drugs, acupuncture, tuina, external application, fumigation（熏蒸）and washing.

　　A. rules　　　　　　B. strategy　　　　　C. measures　　　　D. principle

8) When the secretions become abnormal in amount, color or smell, a _____ activity may be present in the regions or corresponding internal organs.

　　A. ill　　　　　　　B. evil　　　　　　　C. pathological　　　D. pathosis

9) If a disease occurs in the body surface, muscles, or meridians, it is usually regarded as an _____ pattern (affected superficial portion of the body).

A. interior   B. internal   C. external   D. exterior

10) _____ pattern can also be caused by internal damage such as qi stagnation, blood stasis, phlegm obstruction or stagnancy of fluid flow.

A. Superabundant   B. Excess

C. Sufficient   D. Deficient

11) A red _____ is mostly due to the fever of a common cold, or may be a heat pattern due to excessive yang in the *zang-fu* organs.

A. color   B. luster   C. complexion   D. countenance

12) In most cases, wind pathogens are the foremost pathogens to _____ the lung, and they usually join up with cold, heat or dryness pathogens to accomplish the attack.

A. hit   B. strike   C. invade   D. impact

13) Excess of pathogenic qi, with excess manifestations, should be treated by _____.

A. clearing   B. nourishing

C. tonifying   D. purging

14) There is a concept in TCM depicting a _____ disorder primarily affecting brain functions.

A. phlegm   B. sputum   C. dampness   D. water

15) Criteria utilized in making a TCM diagnosis of qi _____ take into account the quality of pain, the area of pain and the response of pain to pressure and temperature.

A. stagnation   B. stasis   C. retention   D. sluggish

Task Three   Translation

Translate the following expressions into English.

1) 四诊   2) 疼痛性质

3) 阳虚   4) 实证

5) 血瘀   6) 气滞

7) 清热泻火   8) 临床表现

9) 治疗原则   10) 诊病

11) 舌苔   12) 腹部触诊

13) 闻诊   14) 标本同治

15) 痰热壅肺   16) 肝气郁结

17) 胀痛   18) 刺痛

19) 胸闷   20) 鉴别诊断

21) 糖尿病患者   22) 主诉

PART Ⅲ TRANSLATION AND WRITING

How to Describe a Pattern

According to traditional Chinese medicine (TCM), each pattern has its etiology(病因) and pathogenesis(病机), which determines the principles and methods of treatment. For the description of a pattern in English, it is recommended that you visit some international websites for further information.

It is commonly recognized that the description of a pattern should usually include the following details: 1) concept of the pattern(证的概念); 2) etiology(病因); 3) pattern analysis(证候分析); 4) the essentials of pattern differentiation(辨证要点); 5) differential diagnosis(鉴别诊断); 6) principles and methods of treatment(治则治法); and 7) representative formula(代表方剂).

The following sentences or expressions are commonly used to describe a pattern.

1) In TCM, the heart blood deficiency is a common pattern due to insufficient heart blood failing to nourish the heart.

中医心血虚证是指心血不足,不能濡养心脏所表现的一种常见证候。

2) Pattern of wind-heat invading lung is usually caused by external invasion of wind-heat.

风热犯肺证多由外感风热所致。

3) The main clinical manifestations of lung-qi deficiency pattern are weak cough, faint low voice, spontaneous sweating, pale complexion, pale tongue and weak pulse.

肺气虚证的主要临床表现有咳嗽无力、语声低怯、自汗、面色苍白、舌质淡、脉虚弱。

4) Deficient spleen-qi fails to lift, leading to the sinking of qi of the middle energizer (*jiao*), and prolapse of the internal organs.

脾气亏虚,升举无力,导致中气下陷、内脏下垂。

5) When water flows over muscles, edema may occur.

水溢肌肤,发为水肿。

6) When static blood accumulates in the body and blocks the meridians and collaterals, there may appear fixed stabbing pain.

瘀血停积于内,经络受阻,则表现为疼痛如针刺,部位固定。

7) When qi gets obstructed by phlegm, leading to unsmooth flow of qi in the chest, chest distress may occur.

气为痰阻,胸中之气不利则胸闷。

8) Liver qi stagnation result in distending pain in the chest and hypochondrium.

肝气郁结可致胸胁胀痛。

9) When pathogenic cold invades the lung, lung qi will fail to diffuse and govern descent and will flow adversely leading to cough, dyspnea, and spitting white sputum.

寒邪客肺,肺失肃降,肺气上逆,导致咳嗽、气喘、咳吐白痰。

10) Red tongue with yellow coating and rapid or slippery pulse are all the manifestations of excessive fire.

舌红苔黄,脉数或滑均为火热炽盛之象。

11) The essentials of pattern differentiation in spleen qi deficiency are poor appetite, abdominal distension, loose stool, and other symptoms of qi deficiency.

脾气虚证辨证要点为食少、腹胀、便溏以及气虚见症。

12) The pattern of blazing liver fire should be considered in the differential diagnosis of liver-yang hyperactivity pattern.

肝火炽盛证应与肝阳上亢证进行鉴别诊断。

13) Yin deficiency pattern is characterized by deficiency-heat, while yang deficiency pattern is characterized by deficiency-cold.

阴虚证以虚热为特点,而阳虚证以虚寒为特点。

14) Heat-clearing method is commonly used in the treatment of heat pattern.

清热法常用于热证的治疗。

15) The representative formula to treat qi deficiency pattern is *Si Junzi* Decoction.

治疗气虚证的代表方剂为四君子汤。

Sample

Kidney-yang Deficiency Pattern

Kidney-yang deficiency is the pattern due to the failure of kidney-yang to warm the body and perform its functions. It is usually caused by congenital yang deficiency, or kidney-yang injury due to excessive sexual activities, old ages, or other chronic diseases.

1) The kidney is located in the lower back and governs the bone, so weakness and cold pain in the lower back and knees will appear because of deficient kidney-yang failing to give warmth. The kidney-yang is recognized as the original yang of the whole body, so the cold body and limbs will appear when kidney-yang loses its warming action. Pale complexion will be present when the deficient yang fails to promote the circulation of qi and blood. And dark complexion will be seen due to severe deficiency of kidney-yang. Deficient yang can't stimulate the spirit, so fatigue (疲乏) occurs. Sex apathy (性冷淡), erectile dysfunction (阳痿) or sterility (不孕不育) also appear because of kidney-yang failing to excite the sexual function. 2) If deficient kidney-yang can't warm the spleen-yang, there occurs chronic diarrhea (腹泻) with undigested food or diarrhea before dawn due to abnormal transportation of the spleen. The disfunction of qi transformation from kidney-yang insufficiency may bring about frequent urination and nocturia (夜尿;遗尿). The insufficient kidney-yang failing to govern the water may cause edema and oliguresis (少尿). The kidney is in the lower energizer (下焦), so the water tends to go down causing more severe edema below the lower back. Enlarged pale tongue with tooth marks and white glossy coating are signals of yang deficiency and retention of water-dampness. The kidney-yang can't motivate the flow of qi and blood, so weak pulse is felt obviously on the

笔记

chi portion of the *cunkou* pulse.

3) The essentials of pattern differentiation in kidney-yang deficiency are weakness and cold pain of the lower back and knees, sex apathy, hypofunction of the body, and other symptoms of yang deficiency.

4) The kidney-yin deficiency pattern should be considered in the differential diagnosis of kidney-yang deficiency pattern. The kidney yin deficiency pattern is characterized by deficiency-heat, while the kidney-yang deficiency pattern is characterized by deficiency-cold.

5) The therapeutic method of warming and tonifying kidney-yang is commonly used in the treatment of kidney- yang deficiency pattern. The representative formula for the kidney-yang deficiency pattern is *Jingui Shenqi* Pill.

Task One Translation

Translate the underlined parts in the above sample into Chinese.

1) _____

_____

2) _____

_____

3) _____

_____

4) _____

_____

5) _____

_____

Task Two Writing

Choose a pattern and write a 200-word description of it. Try to use as many sentence patterns as possible in PART Ⅲ. Alternatively, you may work in pairs on a chosen topic, search the information on the internet, write the introduction and then present it to the class.

_____

_____

_____

PART IV   REFLECTION

Zheng, also known as TCM pattern, is a characteristic profile of all clinical manifestations that can be identified by a TCM practitioner. Clinical treatments of a patient rely on the successful differentiation of a specific *zheng*. Recently, some new technologies and methods such as the systemomics approach (系统组学方法) were introduced in *zheng* research, which significantly facilitates the development of *zheng* theory. A brief introduction to these new technologies and methods and their application in TCM *zheng* differentiation research can be found in journal articles.

Search the internet for information on ***zheng*** and think about the following questions:

1) How do you understand "*zheng*" in TCM and "disease" in Western medicine?

2) Do you see the importance of establishing a research center of *zheng* for the clinical practice?

笔记

Unit 4

Acupuncture-moxibustion and Tuina

LEARNING OUTCOMES

This unit offers you opportunities to:

- **explain** the concepts and functions of acupuncture-moxibustion
- **illustrate** how to manipulate acupuncture-moxibustion and tuina
- **use** the terms related to acupuncture-moxibustion and tuina
- **describe** how to use moxa
- **reflect on** the promotion of acupuncture therapy

PART I   LISTENING AND SPEAKING

Before you listen

In this section you will hear a short passage entitled "The 50th Anniversary of the Broad Use of Acupuncture in the US". The following words and phrases may be of help.

columnist /'kɒləmnɪst/	n.	专栏作家
appendicitis /ə,pendə'saɪtɪs/	n.	阑尾炎
painkiller /'peɪnkɪlə/	n.	止痛药
opioid /'əʊpɪ,ɔɪd/	n.	阿片类药物
session /'seʃ(ə)n/	n.	（针灸等治疗）次数
indigestion /,ɪndɪ'dʒestʃən/	n.	消化不良
fatigue /fə'tiːg/	n.	疲倦
gynecological /,gaɪnəkə'lɒdʒikəl/	a.	妇科的
infertility /,ɪnfəˈtɪlɪti/	n.	不孕
pandemic /pæn'demɪk/	n.	大流行病
accredited /ə'kredɪtɪd/	a.	官方承认的
intermittent /,ɪntə'mɪtənt/	a.	间歇的

While you listen

Listen to the passage carefully and fill in each of the blanks marked from 1) to 10) according to what you have heard.

The 50th Anniversary of the Broad Use of Acupuncture in the US

In 1971, *The New York Times* columnist James Reston opened the door for the treatment in the US. When Reston traveled to China before US President Richard Nixon's visit the following year, he had an acute 1) _____ of appendicitis. While Reston was hospitalized in Beijing, his post-operation pain was treated with acupuncture and moxibustion.

ER-4-1
Listening
practice

His special report "Now, About My Operation in Peking" about his personal experiences and observations on the effectiveness of acupuncture and moxibustion helped 2) _____ the way for the 3) _____ of alternative medicine in the US.

The Chinese medical treatment has been embraced by patients and doctors in the US as an alternative to the powerful painkillers that are behind the widespread 4) _____ of opioids.

In 2020, Medicare, the largest US federal government 5) _____ program,

笔记

79

began covering acupuncture as a treatment for lower back pain due to the nation's opioid 6) _____ . Medicare covers up to 12 sessions in 90 days, with an additional eight sessions in case of improvement for chronic pain.

Many Americans 7) _____ the effect of acupuncture in the treatment of pain, but actually acupuncture is also very good at treating indigestion, gynecological issues like infertility, and mental issues such as insomnia, anxiety and depression. The good thing is that more people are gaining knowledge of acupuncture.

In the COVID-19 pandemic, more and more Americans benefited from acupuncture for their post-COVID conditions, or long COVID, which may be 8) _____ as fatigue, shortness of breath, coughing, cognitive problems, difficulty concentrating, depression, muscle and joint pain, headaches, disorder of smell and taste, rapid heartbeat and intermittent fever, etc.

In the US, as long as anyone completes an accredited educational program and meets the assessments 9) _____ by the National Certification Commission for Acupuncture and Oriental Medicine (NCCAOM) and the state licensing exam, they can 10) _____ work as acupuncturists.

Reference: ZHANG M L. Acupuncture treats post-COVID conditions overseas [EB/OL]. China daily. (2021-09-02) [2022-10-20]. http://www.chinadaily.com.cn/a/202109/02/WS61300d46a310efa1bd66cb5c. html.

After you listen

Please discuss with your partner the following questions and give your presentation to the class.

1) How much do you know about acupuncture?
2) Why can acupuncture work for long COVID and other conditions?

PART II   READING

Text A

Acupuncture and Moxibustion

1   In 1972, an American medical **delegation** observed acupuncture **anesthesia** upon their request to the Chinese Government during the official visit to China with President Richard Nixon. They witnessed Chinese doctors' performing **thoracotomy** and **pneumonectomy** under the surgical light with acupuncture anesthesia only. This was broadcast live by news reporters to the whole world via satellites, leading to an increasing acupuncture enthusiasm in the United States and other Western countries. The magical effect of acupuncture anesthesia made the Americans speak highly of traditional Chinese medicine (TCM), and attracted their great attention to the ancient traditional medical art, acupuncture.

2   Being important components of TCM, acupuncture and moxibustion are some of the most distinctive therapies originated from the early stages of human society in China. In primitive societies, people might have **instinctively** rubbed or **tapped** areas of their bodies in order to **alleviate** pain from injury and disease. Evidence from ancient Chinese medical records and cultural **relics** suggest that treatment with a special stone, *bian* stone, was an **initial** form of acupuncture. In 1963, a 4.5-centimeter-long stone was unearthed at a **Neolithic archaeological** site in **Inner Mongolia,** China. This *bian* stone is believed to be an early medical instrument used to cut **carbuncles** and remove **pus**.

3   With continuous social and technological development, needle materials improved as well. After the introduction of **metallurgy** in the Western Zhou Dynasty (1046 BC–771 BC), metal needles replaced stone. In 1968, four gold and five silver medical needles were found in a Han Dynasty (206 BC–220 AD) tomb. The contemporary needles, made of such materials as gold, silver and **stainless** steel are modeled on the ancient nine needles. To be more specific, the **filiform** needle commonly used at present is made of **durable, elastic** stainless steel that is both non-**corrosive** and inexpensive. Gold, silver or mixed **alloy** needles are expensive, less durable and less elastic, but their **conductivity** is higher, so they are good for warm needling and **electrostimulation**.

4   The acupuncture practitioner treats diseases by stimulating certain points of the body with needles or similar instruments. Since the **shaft** of the filiform needle is slender and flexible, an acupuncturist needs adequate training and practice in needling skills and must develop his finger force in order to make painless insertion and well-skilled manipulation of needles. Finger force practice allows the beginner to develop the pressure needed to **insert** a needle smoothly into the body. Practice may first be conducted on a paper **pad** or cotton ball, which is made by tightly bound multi-folded soft paper or multi-layered cotton **gauze**. The needle should be held with the thumb, **index** and middle fingers of

笔记

one's **dominant** hand **perpendicularly** to the pad or ball. Force is gradually exerted just before the needle tip touches the pad or the ball. After repeated practice, the needle can be inserted smoothly, **dexterously** and rapidly. Then one should practice the commonly used needle **manipulations** on the pad or ball.

5　Needle manipulations are **maneuvers** conducted to promote or regulate the needling **sensation** or arrival of qi (*deqi*). They are classified into basic manipulation and **supplementary** manipulation. The former includes lifting-**thrusting** and **twirling**, while the latter includes pushing, **scraping**, **flicking**, shaking, flying and **vibrating**.

6　Needling sensation, or arrival of qi, refers to a special sensation produced by needling and manipulations. The sensation can be evaluated from two perspectives: that of the patient and that of the acupuncturist. When qi arrives, the acupuncturist can feel tightness around the needle. The patient may have such sensations as soreness, **numbness**, **distention** and heaviness at the point, which may **radiate** along the course of the meridian. If qi does not arrive, the acupuncturist may feel loose around the needle, while the patient may feel nothing.

7　Generally speaking, acupuncture is a relatively safe therapy. However, careless administration, inappropriate manipulation or lack of anatomic knowledge may result in abnormal consequences and even accidents. Acupuncture is **contraindicated** in certain points for pregnant women, infants and patients with spontaneous bleeding or **coagulation** disorders. Caution should be taken when acupuncture is applied to points located close to vital organs.

8　Since acupuncture is often conducted in combination with moxibustion, there is the expression "acupuncture-moxibustion". Moxibustion is a therapy by applying burning **moxa** on acupuncture points. Guided by TCM theory, this therapy aims to **dredge** meridians, regulate qi and blood, keep balance of yin and yang, harmonize the functions of the *zang-fu* organs, and ultimately prevent and treat diseases. Since moxibustion warms the meridians and dissipates cold, it is often used in conditions caused by cold-damp obstruction or pathogenic cold, which are manifested by cold-damp **arthralgia**, **epigastric** pain, **abdominal** pain, **diarrhea** and **dysentery**.

9　Moxa wool made of dried, purified **mugwort** leaves is often shaped into tight, firm **cones**. Their size varies according to the conditions to be treated. A small cone is the size of a grain of wheat; a middle one, the size of a Chinese date **pit**; and a big one, half the size of an **olive**. Cones are **ignited** at the top and placed over the points. Each cone that has burned completely counts as one *zhuang*.

10　In general, moxibustion is applied to the yang meridians first and the yin meridians later, to the upper part first and the lower part later, with fewer and smaller moxa cones first and more and larger moxa cones later.

11　What are the contraindications of moxibustion? Firstly, avoid using moxibustion when treating excess heat patterns or fever due to yin deficiency. Secondly, avoid using scarring moxibustion on the face, **mammary papillae** and areas with large blood vessels.

Finally, avoid using moxibustion on the abdomen and **lumbosacral** region in pregnant women.

12　As integral parts of treatment modalities, acupuncture and moxibustion work to dredge meridians, move qi and activate blood to restore the balance between yin and yang, coordinate the functions of *zang-fu* organs, support healthy qi and eliminate pathogenic factors.

Reference: ZHANG J, ZHAO B X, LAO L X. Acupuncture and moxibustion (International Standard Library of Chinese Medicine) [M]. Beijing: People's Medical Publishing House, 2014.

New words

delegation /ˌdelɪˈgeɪʃn/	n.	a group of people who represent the views of an organization, a country, etc. 代表团
anesthesia /ˌænɪsˈθiːziə/	n.	insensitivity to pain, especially as artificially induced by the administration of gases or the injection of drugs before surgical operations 麻醉
thoracotomy /ˌθɔːrəˈkɔtəmɪ/	n.	surgical incision into the chest wall 开胸手术
pneumonectomy /ˌnjuːmə(ʊ)ˈnektəmɪ/	n.	surgical removal of a lung or part of a lung 肺切除术
instinctively /ɪnˈstɪŋktɪvli/	ad.	without conscious thought; by natural instinct 本能地
tap /tæp/	vt.	hit sb./sth. quickly and lightly 轻敲
alleviate /əˈliːvieɪt/	vt.	make (suffering, deficiency, or a problem) less severe 减轻,缓和
relic /ˈrelɪk/	n.	an object, a tradition, etc. that has survived from a period of time that no longer exists 遗迹
initial /ɪˈnɪʃl/	a.	happening at the beginning 最初的
Neolithic /ˌniːəˈlɪθɪk/	a.	of the latter part of the Stone Age 新石器时代的
archaeological /ˌɑːkiəˈlɔdʒɪk(ə)l/	a.	connected with the study of cultures of the past and of periods of history by examining the remains of buildings and objects found in the ground 考古学的,考古学上的
Inner Mongolia /mɔŋˈgəʊliə/	n.	an autonomous region of northeast China 内蒙古

carbuncle /'kɑ:bʌŋkl/	n.	a large painful swelling under the skin 痈
pus /pʌs/	n.	a thick yellowish or greenish liquid that is produced in an infected wound 脓
metallurgy /mə'tælədʒi/	n.	the scientific study of metals and their uses 冶金学；冶金术
stainless /'steɪnləs/	a.	resistant to discoloration, especially discoloration resulting from corrosion 防锈的
filiform /'faɪlɪfɔ:m/	a.	thread-like 丝状的；线状的；纤维状的
durable /'djʊərəb(ə)l/	a.	likely to last for a long time without breaking or getting weaker 耐用的
elastic /ɪ'læstɪk/	a.	able to stretch and return to its original 有弹性的
corrosive /kə'rəʊsɪv/	a.	tending to destroy sth. slowly by chemical action 腐蚀性的
alloy /'ælɔɪ/	n.	a metal that is formed by mixing two types of metal together, or by mixing metal with another substance 合金
conductivity /ˌkɒndʌk'tɪvəti/	n.	ability to conduct electricity, heat, etc. 传导性
electrostimulation /iˌlektrəˌstimju'leiʃən/	n.	electrical stimulation of a nerve, muscle, etc. 电刺激
shaft /ʃɑ:ft/	n.	a long thin piece of wood or metal that forms part of a spear axe, golf club, or other object 柄；杆
insert /ɪn's3:t/	vt.	put sth. into sth. else 插入
pad /pæd/	n.	a thick piece of soft material that is used, for example, for absorbing liquid, cleaning or protecting sth. 软垫
gauze /gɔ:z/	n.	a type of thin cotton cloth used for covering and protecting wounds 纱布
index /'ɪndeks/ (finger)	n.	the finger next to the thumb 食指
dominant /'dɒmɪnənt/	a.	having power and influence over others 占优势的；占支配地位的
perpendicular /ˌp3:pən'dɪkjələ/	a.	forming an angle of 90° with another line or surface 垂直的
dexterously /'dekstrəsli/	ad.	in a way that shows the ability to perform a difficult action quickly and skillfully with the hands 灵巧地

manipulation /mə,nɪpjʊ'leɪʃ(ə)n/	n.	the action of manipulating sth. in a skillful manner（熟练的）操作，操纵
maneuver /mə'nʊvə/	n.	a movement performed with care and skill 谨慎而熟练的动作
sensation /sen'seɪʃn/	n.	a feeling that you get when sth. affects your body 感觉；知觉
supplementary /,sʌplɪ'mentri/	a.	provided in addition to sth. else in order to improve or complete it 补充的；额外的
thrust /θrʌst/	vt.	push a pointed object into sb./sth. with a sudden strong movement 插；戳
twirl /twɜːl/	vt.	spin quickly and lightly round, especially repeatedly 捻转
scrape /skreɪp/	vt.	remove sth. from a surface by moving sth. sharp and hard like a knife across it 刮
flick /flɪk/	vt.	hit sth. with a sudden quick movement, especially using your finger and thumb together, or your hand 轻弹；轻拍
vibrate /vaɪ'breɪt/	vt.	make sth. move from side to side very quickly and with small movements 使振动；使颤动
numbness /'nʌmnəs/	n.	a lack of feeling in a part of the body 无感觉；麻木
distention /dɪs'tenʃən/	n.	the state of being stretched beyond normal dimensions 膨胀；延伸
radiate /'reɪdieɪt/	vi.	(of light, heat, or other energy) be emitted in the form of rays or waves 辐射；发散
contraindicate /,kɒntrə'ɪndɪkeɪt/	vt.	advise against or indicate the possible danger of a drug, treatment, etc. 对……禁忌，（药物或疗法）禁用于
coagulation /kəʊ,æɡjʊ'leɪʃn/	n.	the process of a liquid becoming thick and partly solid 凝结、凝血
moxa /'mɒksə/	n.	a soft woolly mass prepared from the ground young leaves of a Eurasian Artemisia 艾
dredge /dredʒ/	vt.	clear the bed of (a harbor, river, or other area of water) by scooping out mud, weeds, and rubbish with a dredge 疏通，清淤（河道等）

笔记

85

arthralgia /ɑːˈθrældʒə/	*n.*	pain in a joint 关节痛
epigastric /ˌepɪˈgæstrɪk/	*a.*	of or relating to the anterior walls of the abdomen 胃脘部的，上腹部的
abdominal /æbˈdɔmɪn(ə)l/	*a.*	relating to or connected with the abdomen 腹部的
diarrhea /ˌdaɪəˈrɪə/	*n.*	an illness in which waste matter is emptied from the bowels much more frequently than normal, and in liquid form 腹泻
dysentery /ˈdɪsəntri/	*n.*	an infection of the bowels that causes severe diarrhea with loss of blood 痢疾
mugwort /ˈmʌgwəːt/	*n.*	a plant of the daisy family, with aromatic divided leaves that are dark green above and whitish below, native to north temperate regions 艾蒿
cone /kəʊn/	*n.*	a solid or hollow object with a round flat base and sides that slope up to a point 圆锥体
pit /pɪt/	*n.*	the large hard seed of a fruit or vegetable 核
olive /ˈɔlɪv/	*n.*	a small green or black fruit with a strong taste, used in cooking and for its oil 橄榄
ignite /ɪgˈnaɪt/	*vt.*	cause to catch fire 点燃
mammary /ˈmæməri/	*a.*	connected with the breasts 乳房的；乳腺的
papillae /pəˈpɪli/	*n.*	a small nipple-shaped protuberance 乳头状突起
lumbosacral /ˌlʌmbəʊˈseɪkrəl/	*a.*	of or relating to the loins and sacrum 腰骶的

Phrases and expressions

acupuncture anesthesia	针刺麻醉
speak highly of sth.	高度赞扬
alleviate pain	缓解疼痛
initial form	雏形，最初形式
Neolithic archaeological site	新石器时代考古遗址
remove pus	排脓
filiform needle	毫针

stainless steel	不锈钢
cotton gauze	纱布辅料
index finger	食指
dominant hand	惯用手,优势手
needling sensation	得气
dredge meridians	疏通经络
cold-damp obstruction	寒湿痹阻
epigastric pain	胃脘痛
abdominal pain	腹痛
scarring moxibustion	瘢痕灸
lumbosacral region	腰骶部

Task One　Preview

1. Learn the following roots and affixes. Write out the Chinese meaning of the given words.

Roots/ Affixes	Meaning of roots/affixes	Words	Chinese meaning of the given words
anethes (o)	insensitivity	anesthesia	_____
		anesthetic	_____
arch-	ancient	archaeology	_____
		archaic	_____
-bustion	burning	combustion	_____
		moxibustion	_____
carb	carbon	carbuncle	_____
		bicarbonate	_____
-cular	pertaining to	retinacular	_____
		spiracular	_____
dext	the right-hand side	ambidextrous	_____
		dexterously	_____
-ectomy	removal	thoracotomy	_____
		pneumonectomy	_____
electro	electricity	electrostimulation	_____
		electrosurgery	_____
fil (i)	thread	filament	_____
		filiform	_____
lithic	stone	neolithic	_____
		paleolithic	_____

笔记

mani-/manu	hand	manipulate	_____
		manual	_____
pend	hang	perpendicular	_____
		pendulum	_____
puncture	prick	arteriopuncture	_____
		colopuncture	_____
radi (o)	radiating	radiance	_____
		radiotherapy	_____
thorac (o)	thorax	thoracoplasty	_____
		thoracoscope	_____
-uncle	little, small	peduncle	_____
		siphuncle	_____
urgy	technology	metallurgy	_____
		micrurgy	_____
vibr	swing	vibrate	_____
		revibrate	_____

2. Write down the questions you would like to ask or discuss about the text.

_____

_____

_____

Task Two　Speaking

1. Answer the following questions according to the text.

1) What led to an increasing acupuncture enthusiasm in the United States and other Western countries in 1972?

2) What was an initial form of acupuncture instrument?

3) Presently, what is the commonly-used filiform needle made of?

4) What is the classification of needle manipulations?

5) What will acupuncturists and patients feel when there is needling sensation?

6) What are the contraindications of acupuncture therapy?

7) How do you define moxibustion therapy? What are its suitable indications?

8) What is the sequence of applying moxibustion on the body?

2. Work in pairs or groups and exchange views on the following news.

Guidelines on Acupuncture and Moxibustion

Intervention for COVID-19

　　It is known that many therapeutic methods of traditional Chinese medicine (TCM), e.g., Chinese herbal decoction, acupuncture, moxibustion, acupoint plaster, auricular acupuncture and cupping, have been employed in the treatment for COVID-19. In the regions where TCM therapeutic modalities were utilized, the curative rate increased, the number of severe cases decreased and higher hospital discharge rate was found. At present the TCM intervention has effectively blocked the spread of COVID-19 in China.

In response to the Chinese government's call upon the solidarity in the fight against COVID-19 and in order to better apply TCM external therapies to the prevention and treatment for COVID-19, China Association of Acupuncture–Moxibustion (CAAM) developed and issued the *Guidelines on Acupuncture and Moxibustion Intervention for COVID-19* (2nd edition) (hereinafter *Guidelines*).The *Guidelines* is established to assist the application of TCM techniques, e.g., acupuncture and moxibustion in the treatment for COVID-19. The therapeutic methods of each stage are introduced as follows:

1. Acupuncture–moxibustion intervention at the medical observation stage (for suspected cases): The patients are needed to activate healthy qi and the functions of the lung and the spleen, and to expel pestilential factors to strengthen the defensive capacity of their internal organs. Acupoints selected are as follows: Group 1: Fengmen (BL12), Feishu (BL13), and Pishu (BL20); Group 2: Hegu (LI4), Quchi (LI11), Chize (LU5) and Yuji (LU10); Group 3: Qihai (CV6), Zusanli (ST36) and Sanyinjiao (SP6). One or two acupoints are selected from each group in one treatment.

2. Acupuncture–moxibustion intervention at the treatment stage (for confirmed cases): The patients are needed to activate the functions of the lung and the spleen, protect internal organs, reduce impairment, eliminate pestilential factors, promote earth (spleen) to generate metal (lung), prevent deterioration, reduce stress and boost confidence against the illness. Acupoints selected are as follows: Group 1: Hegu (LI4), Taichong (LR3), Tiantu (CV22), Chize (LU5), Kongzui (LU6), Zusanli (ST36) and Sanyinjiao (SP6); Group 2: Dazhu (BL11), Fengmen (BL12), Feishu (BL13), Xinshu (BL15) and Geshu (BL17); Group 3: Zhongfu (LU1), Danzhong (CV17), Qihai (CV6), Guanyuan (CV4) and Zhongwan (CV12). For mild or common cases, 2 or 3 acupoints are selected from Group 1 or Group 2 in each treatment. For severe cases, 2 or 3 acupoints are selected from Group 3.

3. Acupuncture-moxibustion intervention at the recovery stage: The patients are needed to clear the residual pestilential factors, promote the repairment of internal organs, and restore healthy qi and the functions of the lung and the spleen. Acupoints selected are as follows: Neiguan (PC6), Zusanli (ST36), Zhongwan (CV12), Tianshu (ST25) and Qihai (CV6).

Reference: LIU W H, GUO S N, WANG F, et al. Understanding of guidance for acupuncture and moxibustion interventions on COVID-19 (second edition) issued by CAAM [J]. World journal of acupuncture-moxibustion, 2020, 30 (1): 1-4.

Topic for discussion: Discuss the treatment mechanism of the acupoints selected for the mild or common cases.

Task Three　Vocabulary

1. Match up each word in Column A with its appropriate definition from Column B.

Column A	Column B
1) anesthesia	a. pain in a joint
2) thoracotomy	b. hit sth. with a sudden quick movement
3) pneumonectomy	c. loose, watery stools three or more times a day
4) carbuncle	d. spin quickly and lightly round, especially repeatedly
5) pus	e. an infection of the bowels that causes severe diarrhea with loss of blood
6) arthralgia	f. a large painful swelling under the skin
7) diarrhea	g. the action of manipulating sth. in a skillful manner
8) dysentery	h. make sth. move from side to side very quickly and with small movements
9) lumbosacral	i. insensitivity to pain
10) manipulation	j. a thick yellowish or greenish liquid that is produced in an infected wound
11) thrust	k. surgical removal of a lung or part of a lung
12) twirl	l. surgical incision into the chest wall
13) flick	m. push a pointed object into sb./sth. with a sudden strong movement
14) vibrate	n. of or relating to the loins and sacrum

2. Fill in the blanks with the words given below. Change the form where necessary.

refer to	proportional	stimulate	rebalance	associate with
stand for	base on	subtle	restore	along
recognize	calculate	palpate	remarkable	activate

Acupuncture Points

Acupuncture points (also called acupoints) are the specific locations on the body surface for diagnostic detection and therapeutic stimulation. In traditional Chinese medicine (TCM), several hundred acupuncture points are claimed to be located 1)_____ what practitioners call meridians. There are also numerous "extra points" not 2)_____ a particular meridian.

TCM theory for the selection of such points and their effectiveness is that they work by 3)_____ the meridian system to bring about relief by 4)_____ yin, yang and qi. This theory is 5)_____ the paradigm of TCM and has no analogue (相

似物)in Western medicine.

Body acupoints are generally located using a measurement unit, called *cun*, which is calibrated (校准) according to their 6)_____ distances from various landmark points on the body. Acupoint location usually depends on specific anatomical landmarks that can be 7)_____.

Points tend to be located where nerves enter a muscle, the midpoint of the muscle, or at the enthesis (起止点) where the muscle joins with the bone. Location by palpation for tenderness is also a common way of locating acupoints. Points may also be located by feeling for 8)_____ differences in temperature on the skin surface or over the skin surface, as well as changes in the tension or "stickiness" of the skin and tissue.

Body acupoints are referred to either by their traditional name, or by the name of the meridian on which they are located, followed by a number to indicate what order the point is in the meridian. A common point on the hand, for example, is named Hegu, and 9)_____ as LI4, which means that it is the fourth point on the Large Intestine Meridian. According to WHO standard, 361 meridian points and 48 extra points are generally 10)_____, but the number of points has changed over the centuries.

Task Four   Translation

1. Study the following sentences and pay attention to the underlined parts.

1) The magical effect of acupuncture anesthesia made the Americans speak highly of TCM. (para. 1)

2) The needles of today, made of such materials as gold, silver and stainless steel are modeled on the ancient nine needles. (para. 3)

3) Finger force practice allows the beginner to develop the pressure needed to insert a needle smoothly into the body. (para. 4)

4) They are classified into basic manipulation and supplementary manipulation. The former includes lifting-thrusting and twirling; the latter includes pushing, scraping, flicking, shaking, flying and vibrating. (para. 5)

5) Caution should be taken when acupuncture is applied to points located close to vital organs. (para. 7)

6) Moxa wool made of dried, purified mugwort leaves is often shaped into tight, firm cones. Their size varies according to the condition to be treated. (para. 9)

2. Translate the following sentences into English.

1) 非洲国家政党和人士高度评价中国采取具体措施,帮助他们抗击新型冠状病毒感染疫情,为非洲国家战胜疫情增添了信心。

2) 现代针灸中,最常见的是不锈钢制成的毫针。针灸针也可以由银或金制成。

3) 当经络通道打开时,气随之进入人体组织器官。

4) 针刺手法分为基本手法和辅助手法，前者包括提插和捻转，后者包括循法、刮法、弹法、摇法、飞法、震颤法等。

5) 艾条点燃时非常热，因此必须小心，防止灼伤患者皮肤。

6) 为缓慢产生强热量，艾绒被制成非常紧实的圆锥形艾炷，其大小根据治疗需要而异。

Text B

Gunfa (Rolling Manipulation)

1　*Gunfa*[1] is one of the hardest techniques to master and it takes time and practice to get right. *Gunfa* can be applied in a very focused way to one particular area such as the shoulder joint, or moved gradually along a meridian or section of a meridian. It can be accompanied by passive movements[2] of a joint, particularly the neck and shoulder.

2　The area or side of the body you are working on will **dictate** which hand would be best to use. *Gunfa* can also be applied with both hands working simultaneously. This is most common when working down the Bladder Meridian on the back.

How to practice *gunfa*

3　*Gunfa* must be practiced on a sand bag before attempting to apply it to a human body. It will take about 3–4 months of daily practice to get to grips with it on the sand bag, and a further 6 months to begin to feel really comfortable and competent with the technique.

Starting position

4　Put your sand bag on a table in front of you and slightly to one side. The table should not be too high; you need to feel that you can relax the weight of your arm down onto the sand bag. If you are practicing with your right hand, place the bag slightly to your right; this will give you enough space to allow your elbow and upper arm to swing freely.

5　Stand with your feet shoulder width apart and knees slightly bent, or in a forward **lunge** posture.[3] Place your little finger **knuckle** onto the sand bag, fingers relaxed and loosely curled. Imagine your knuckle is glued to the spot (some students find it helpful to mark a spot on the bag). The little finger knuckle is the **pivotal** point and never leaves the spot.

Step one— Rolling out

6　Initiating the movement from your elbow, rotate your forearm and extend your wrist, rolling the triangular area between your fifth and third knuckles and the head of your **ulna** onto the sand bag smoothly and evenly. Keep rolling out until your wrist is fully extended,

---

① 　*Gunfa*:（推拿）㨰法，亦可意译为 rolling manipulation (maneuver)。
② 　passive movements: 被动运动，是指患者肌肉放松，完全依靠外力帮助来完成的运动。
③ 　forward lunge posture: 弓箭步，即前腿弓、后腿直的前弓箭步姿势。

palm facing upwards, fingers extended but relaxed. Your elbow and upper arm should now be out, away from the side of your body.

Step two— Rolling back

7   Keeping the little finger knuckle glued to the spot, bring your elbow and upper arm back to your side allowing your wrist to straighten and the back of your hand to roll off the sand bag back to the starting position.

8   Initially, practice for 10 minutes each day, 5 minutes with each hand. Let your dominant hand[①] teach your nondominant hand. Start slowly and get it technically correct.

9   Apply the natural weight of your arm plus a little more. Do not add too much pressure at the start of practice— just enough to make you feel securely in place. Remember that the rolling movement does not start in your hand. It is your elbow and the extensor muscles of your forearm that propel and power the movement. When observed from behind, the elbow should look like a chicken's wing **rhythmically** moving back and forth. Think of your hand as a **greasy** metal ball rolling smoothly with constant even pressure.

10   Build your practice up to 20 minutes per day, and after 2 or 3 months, your wrist will be more flexible and your muscles stronger. At this stage you can begin to practice on the human body. Ideally, practice on fellow students, colleagues, friends and family and try applying *gunfa* to a variety of areas. As you become more competent, gradually use your body weight to add more pressure to the area you are treating. Build up your speed bit by bit to the **optimum** 120–160 cycles per minute.

Suggestion for practice on a volunteer

11   We suggest you start by practicing on the lower back, focusing your technique on one area such as around Shenshu (BL23) for several minutes and then gradually moving down the Bladder Meridian, over the **buttock** and down the leg to the ankle. Once you have arrived at the ankle, **swap** hands and work your way back up to the lower back. When using *gunfa* to move from one place to another like this, the little finger knuckle acts as a guide focusing the technique along the meridian and on any specific points that require attention along the way.

12   With your volunteer sitting in a chair, apply *gunfa* around Fengchi (GB20) in a focused manner, then try moving from here down to Jianjing (GB21). You will need to hold his/her head with your other hand and gently **tilt** it away from the side you are working on. This is an example of *gunfa* plus passive movement. Repeat on the other side.

13   Also in the sitting position apply *gunfa* to the shoulder joint. Hold the volunteer's arm around the elbow with your other hand, keeping his/her forearm close to your body. This will help to support his/her arm properly and keep you in a good position for applying passive movement to the joint.

14   If you are working on your volunteer's left shoulder, stand facing his/her back, hold his/her arm with your left hand and apply *gunfa* all around the posterior aspect of the joint.

---

① dominant hand: 惯用手,优势手,多数人为右手。而 nondominant hand 即是指非惯用手,多数人为左手。

Standing in a forward lunge and moving from your *Dantian*,[①] rock forward and back to create some simple passive movement or twist and rotate his/her arm to expose more of the Triple Energizer[②] and Small Intestine Meridians. Then move around to work on the anterior aspect of the joint. Now your left arm applies *gunfa* and the right arm the passive movements. From this position, twist and rotate to expose the Lung Meridian.

15　Watch out for the following common mistakes that can develop during the initial months of practice:

- Incorrect hand positioning.
- Driving the movement from the wrist rather than from the relaxed free movement of the elbow and forearm.
- The technique becomes **jerky** rather than smooth usually from adding too much pressure too soon.
- The pressure is uneven, usually too strong rolling out and too weak rolling back.
- The technique is too light and superficial rubbing back and forth over the skin surface.

Clinical application and therapeutic effects

16　*Gunfa* is generally applied to large muscular areas, shoulders, back, waist, buttocks, hips, arms and legs. It can be used to stimulate points when applied in a very focused manner. It is often used along the course of the meridian **sinews** and the primary meridian pathways. It can also be applied to the abdomen and the **pectoral** muscles of the chest.

17　*Gunfa* has a deep, penetrating and warming effect. It can be used effectively to move through from the **adaptive** to the **analgesic** level of treatment. In this case the application starts gently, relatively superficially and at a moderate pace. Gradually over a period of 5–10 minutes it becomes increasingly deeper and more driven, building in pace.

18　*Gunfa* dredges the meridians, clearing pathogenic wind, cold and dampness. It promotes the circulation of qi and blood and removes stasis. It relaxes **tendons** and muscles, helps to break up **adhesions**, alleviates pain and muscle **spasms**, reduces swelling and **lubricates** joints.

Common uses

19　Use *gunfa* for any type of *Bi* pattern[③], any meridian sinew[④] problems such as muscular pain and **stiffness**, soft tissue injuries and repetitive strain injury (RSI).[⑤] Use it for back pain and **sciatica**, frozen shoulder and tennis elbow.

20　*Gunfa* is an essential technique in the treatment of *Wei* pattern[⑥] including stroke

---

① *Dantian*: 丹田，道家修炼及气功意守之处，此处应指下丹田（脐下 3 寸关元穴处）。

② Triple Energizer: 三焦，亦可音译为 *Sanjiao*。世界卫生组织（Standard Acupuncture Nomenclature: Part 1）（1991 年）和我国国家标准均将 "三焦" 译作 Triple Energizer。

③ *Bi* pattern: 痹证。

④ meridian sinew: 经筋，亦有译作 meridian tendon。

⑤ repetitive strain injury (RSI): 重复性劳损，指因长时间重复使用某组肌肉造成的损害。

⑥ *Wei* pattern: 痿证，亦有译作 atrophy-flaccidity syndrome 或 *Wei*–flaccidity pattern。

笔记

sequelae[1] and all forms of **paralysis** and dysfunction of the motor nerves[2]. Use it for any case that involves numbness in the limbs. Besides, it is also very effective as part of treatment for abdominal pain with fullness and distension caused by qi stagnation.

Reference: PRITCHARD S. Tuina— a manual of Chinese massage therapy [M]. London: Chullchill Livingstone (Elsevier), 2010:19-22.

New Words

dictate /dɪkˈteɪt/	*vt.*	control or decisively affect; determine 支配,决定
lunge /lʌn(d)ʒ/	*n.*	the basic attacking move in fencing, in which the leading foot is thrust forward close to the floor with the knee bent while the back leg remains straightened 前腿弯曲后腿蹬直的弓箭步（击剑）
knuckle /ˈnʌk(ə)l/	*n.*	part of a finger at a joint where the bone is near the surface, especially where the finger joins the hand 指关节
pivotal /ˈpɪvətl/	*a.*	fixed on or as if on a pivot 枢轴的
ulna /ˈʌlnə/	*n.*	(*pl.* ulnae; ulnas) the thinner and longer of the two bones in the human forearm, on the side opposite to the thumb 尺骨
rhythmically /ˈrɪðmɪkli/	*ad.*	in a rhythmic manner 有节奏地
greasy /ˈgriːsi/	*a.*	covered with, resembling, or produced by grease or oil 油腻的
optimum /ˈɔptɪməm/	*a.*	most conducive to a favorable outcome; best 最适宜的,最佳的
buttock /ˈbʌtək/	*n.*	either of the two round fleshy parts of the human body that form the bottom 臀部
swap /swɔp/	*vt.*	take part in an exchange of 交换
tilt /tɪlt/	*vt.*	cause to move into a sloping position 使倾斜
jerky /ˈdʒəːki/	*a.*	characterized by abrupt stops and starts 忽动忽停的
sinew /ˈsɪnjuː/	*n.*	a piece of tough fibrous tissue uniting muscle to bone 肌腱

---

① stroke sequelae: 脑卒中后遗症,亦有译作 sequela of apoplexy 或 sequela of cerebrovascular accident (CVA)。

② motor nerve: 运动神经。

pectoral /'pekt(ə)r(ə)l/	a.	relating to the breast or chest 胸部的
adaptive /ə'dæptɪv/	a.	characterized by or given to adaptation 适应的，有适应能力的
analgesic /ˌæn(ə)l'dʒi:zɪk/	a.	(of a drug) acting to relieve pain 止痛的
tendon /'tendən/	n.	a flexible but inelastic（无弹性的）cord of strong fibrous collagen tissue attaching a muscle to a bone 肌腱
adhesion /əd'hi:ʒən/	n.	an abnormal adhering of surfaces due to inflammation or injury 粘连
spasm /'spæz(ə)m/	n.	a sudden involuntary muscular contraction or convulsive movement 痉挛；抽搐
lubricate /'lu:brɪkeɪt/	vt.	apply a substance such as oil or grease to (an engine or component) so as to minimize friction and allow smooth movement 使润滑
stiffness /'stɪfnəs/	n.	inability to move easily and without pain 僵硬，强直
sciatica /saɪ'ætɪkə/	n.	pain in the back, hip and outer side of the leg, caused by pressure on the sciatic nerve 坐骨神经痛
sequela /sɪ'kwi:lə/	n.	(*pl.* sequelae) a condition which is the consequence of a previous disease or injury 后遗症
paralysis /pə'rælɪsɪs/	n.	the loss of the ability to move (and sometimes to feel anything) in part or most of the body, typically as a result of illness, poison, or injury 瘫痪，麻痹

Phrases and expressions

get right	清楚无误地了解
get to grips with	对付；掌握要领
pivotal point	轴心，中心点
in place	在恰当的位置
extensor muscle	伸肌
posterior aspect	后侧
watch out	当心
at a moderate pace	以适度的速度
frozen shoulder	五十肩，冻结肩

tennis elbow	网球肘
qi stagnation	气滞

Task One   Preview

1. Learn the following roots and affixes. Write out the Chinese meaning of the given words.

Roots/ Affixes	Meaning of roots/affixes	Words	Chinese meaning of the given words
angi (o)	of blood vessel	angiocardiography	_____
		angiotensin	_____
arteri (o)	of the artery	arteriostenosis	_____
		endoarteritis	_____
cerebr (o)	of the brain	cerebroaphy	_____
		cerebromeningitis	_____
cortic (o)	of the adrenal or cerebral cortices	corticosteroid	_____
		corticomotoneuron	_____
crani (o)	relating to the cranium	craniocerebral	_____
		craniomandibular	_____
cyst (o)	of the urinary bladder	cystitis	_____
		cystoscopy	_____
dict	say, assert	dictate	_____
		dictator	_____
femor (o)	relating to the thigh bone	femorotibial	_____
		femoropopliteal	_____
hidr (o)	perspiration, sweating	anhidrosis	_____
		hyperhidrosis	_____
ischi (o)	of ischium or hucklebone	ischiatitis	_____
		ischiococcygeal	_____
mast (o)	mammary	mastitis	_____
		mastocarcinoma	_____
myel (o)	relating to the marrow of brain and bone	myelofibrosis	_____
		myelencephalitis	_____
oesophag (o)	esophageal	oesophagitis	_____
		esophagospasm	_____
phobia	an extreme or irrational fear of or aversion to sth.	photophobia	_____
		hydrophobia	_____

笔记

pseud (o)-	not genuine; sham	pseudoacusia	_____
		pseudoarthrosis	_____
rect (o)	of the rectum	rectoscopy	_____
		rectostenosis	_____
sclerosis	a hardening of tissue and other anatomical features	artherosclerosis	_____
		fibrosclerosis	_____
tonsill (o)	of the tonsil	tonsillitis	_____
		tonsillectomy	_____

2. Write down the questions you would like to ask or discuss about the text.

_____

_____

_____

Task Two   Vocabulary

Choose the word or phrase that can best complete the statements.

1) Poor nutrition in the early stages of infancy can _____ adult growth.

   A. degenerate   B. deteriorate   C. boost   D. retard

2) She had a terrible accident, but _____ she wasn't killed.

   A. at all events   B. in the long run

   C. at large   D. in vain

3) His weak chest _____ him to winter illness.

   A. predicts   B. predisposes   C. prevails   D. preoccupies

4) The _____ conditions and places are likely to cause diseases.

   A. unsanitary   B. insidious   C. insane   D. inefficacious

5) All instruments that come into contact with the patient must be _____ before being used by others.

   A. quarantined   B. labeled   C. sterilized   D. retained

6) Humor can also be a powerful _____ against stress and misfortune.

   A. bravery   B. blossom   C. buffet   D. buffer

7) The muscular _____ can affect the way we feel mentally.

   A. potency   B. fiber   C. lethargy   D. synthesis

8) There are over 200 acupuncture points on the outer ear alone which _____ different parts of the body, and placing needles in these points might help specific conditions.

   A. respond to   B. correspond to   C. relate with   D. reflect on

9) We _____ that diet is related to most types of cancer but we don't have definite proof.

   A. suspend   B. supervise   C. suspect   D. supervene

10) A patient who is dying of incurable cancer of the throat is in terrible pain, which can no longer be satisfactorily _____.

    A. alleviated   B. abolished   C. demolished   D. diminished

11) She is admitted to the hospital with complaints of upper abdominal pain and _____ for fatty foods.

    A. preference   B. persistence   C. intolerance   D. appetence

12) Doctors are concerned with health of people from _____ to the grave.

    A. perception   B. reception   C. deception   D. conception

13) Her dietician thought that _____ diet and moderate exercise would help her recover soon.

    A. temporary   B. temperate   C. tentative   D. tempting

14) The great risk for rickets is in _____ breastfed infants who are not supplemented with 400 IU of Vitamin D a day.

    A. exceptionally   B. practically

    C. exclusively   D. proportionately

15) Despite the limitations of a standard CT, it does a _____ job of picturing the internal anatomy of the body.

    A. supreme   B. superb   C. sufficient   D. superfluous

Task Three   Translation

Translate the following expressions into English.

    1) 针灸疗法   2) 经络系统

    3) 针刺麻醉   4) 针刺感应

    5) 拔罐疗法   6) 奇穴

    7) 提插   8) 捻转

    9) 耳针疗法   10) 自发性出血倾向

    11) 凝血障碍   12) 瘢痕灸

    13) 毫针   14) 艾炷

    15) 肌肉痉挛   16) 电刺激

    17) 针灸干预   18) 替代医学

    19) 酸胀沉麻   20) 经穴

笔记

PART Ⅲ   TRANSLATION AND WRITING

How to Use Moxa

Moxa sticks are made from the leaves of a plant (Artemisia vulgaris). Moxibustion is the burning of moxa herbal preparation and used to stimulate meridians and acupuncture points. The intention of using this heat therapy is to warm and invigorate the flow of qi in the body and dispel certain pathogenic influences.

Instructions for the use of moxa usually include the following details: 1) when to use moxa (何时使用); 2) what should be prepared (准备用具); 3) how to use moxa (如何施灸); 4) duration of moxa treatment (灸疗时长); and 5) safety issue (安全问题).

The following sentences or expressions are commonly used to give instructions of using moxa.

1) Moxa should only ever be used according to the instructions given to you by your doctor. If in doubt, don't use it until you have consulted him/her.

只有医生允许才能用艾灸。如不确定，咨询医生之后再用。

2) Moxibustion is used for pain due to injury or arthritis, especially in "cold" patterns where the pain naturally feels better with the application of heat.

艾灸用于因受伤或关节炎导致的疼痛，特别是得热则舒的"寒证"。

3) In addition to a stick of moxa, you will probably need a large ashtray or small bowl filled with some sand or dry dirt, a candle and matches, or a cigarette lighter.

除了艾条，你可能会需要一个大的烟灰缸或装满沙子或干燥泥土的小碗、蜡烛、火柴或打火机。

4) Light the end of the moxa stick with the candle or the cigarette lighter.

用蜡烛或打火机点燃艾条末端。

5) Once lit, gently blow on the tip to make it glow. Be careful about flying embers.

艾条点燃后，轻轻吹其顶端让艾条燃红。当心飞起的余烬伤人。

6) Pay attention. Don't burn yourself.

注意，切勿烫伤自己。

7) The glowing end of the moxa stick is held over specific areas, often corresponding to certain acupuncture points.

把点燃的艾条悬灸于人体特定部位，这些部位通常对应某些穴位。

8) The smoldering moxa stick is held about an inch or two above the surface of the skin until the area reddens and becomes suffused with warmth.

把燃烧着的艾条悬灸于体表上方大约1-2英寸之处，直到该部位泛红、发热。

9) Take periodic breaks from warming your body to clear off the loose ash from the end of the stick.

定时暂停艾灸，移开艾条，清除艾灸灰烬。

10) You can gently tap or scrape the ash several times on the rim of your ashtray so

that any loose ash is knocked off.

可以在烟灰缸边缘轻叩或轻刮几次艾条,以便敲落艾灰。

11) After a few seconds the moxa stick will need to be moved regularly or you will eventually burn the skin surface.

每隔几秒,即需移开艾条,否则皮肤表面终会被烫伤。

12) The best way to move the stick is either in small circles or with a "pecking" motion up and down every couple of seconds.

移动艾条最好的方式是画小圆圈或如小鸟啄食般,每隔数秒上下移动。

13) If the skin starts to get too hot, back the moxa stick off further from the skin or stop for a few seconds before continuing.

如果感觉太烫,将艾条燃端离肌肤再远一些,或稍停几秒再继续。

14) Covering the burning end entirely in sand or dirt is the best way to extinguish the moxa stick.

熄灭艾条最好的方法是将整个艾条燃端全部没入沙土里捻灭。

15) Moxa should be applied according to your practitioner's instructions, generally five to ten minutes per point or area.

施灸应当遵照医嘱,通常每个穴位或部位灸 5~10 分钟。

Sample

Instructions for the Use of the Moxa Stick

Simply light one end with a cigarette lighter or hold over a candle. With smokeless moxa it may take several minutes to light but when the stick is correctly lit, you will be able to hold the lit end two to three centimeters from the dorsum of your hand and feel pleasant radiating warmth.

1) Hold the lit end of the stick over the area to be treated, maintaining a distance of at least two to three centimeters so that there is never any direct contact with the skin. The moxa stick is then moved slowly over the area being treated, and the area will start to feel pleasantly warm. 2) When moxa is used to turn a breech or posterior positioned fetus, the therapeutic time is 20 minutes for bilateral points respectively. During this time, the moxibustion by bird-pecking technique is applicable on the point Zhiyin (BL67). 3) Moxibustion with moxa stick on other acupuncture points may be applied on each point for five to seven minutes or until the area become tolerant but comfortable hot.

Make sure the moxa stick remains hot. Re-light if there is no radiating warmth. 4) Never touch the lighted end of a moxa stick even if it no longer appears to be glowing.

When treatment has finished, place the moxa stick in a glass jar lined with dry rice to prevent the heat cracking the glass bottom. 5) When the lid is screwed on firmly, the moxa stick is deprived of oxygen and cannot continue to burn.

Task One　Translation

Translate the underlined parts in the above sample into Chinese.

1) _____

_____

2) _____

_____

3) _____

_____

4) _____

_____

5) _____

_____

Task Two　Writing

　　Choose a TCM therapy and write a 200-word instruction for the use of it. Try to use as many sentence patterns as possible in PART Ⅲ. Alternatively, you may work in pairs on a chosen topic, search the information on the internet, write the instruction and then present it to the class.

_____

_____

_____

_____

_____

_____

PART IV   REFLECTION

A study shows that acupuncture may provide some allergy relief, but researchers say a placebo effect may be responsible for some improvement. Experts suggest that more researches need to be conducted on the issue. Please read the article "Acupuncture may be antidote for allergies" available at http://edition.cnn.com/2013/02/19/health/acpuncture-allergies/ and think about the following questions:

1) What are the obstacles for Westerners to accept acupuncture therapy?

2) Which is more important in convincing Westerners to accept acupuncture therapy, scientific proof or clinical effectiveness?

笔记

Disease Prevention and Treatment in Traditional Chinese Medicine

LEARNING OUTCOMES

This unit offers you opportunities to:

- **explain** the role of traditional Chinese medicine (TCM) in preventing and treating diseases
- **evaluate** emotional factors in people's health
- **make** suggestions from a TCM perspective
- **use** the terms related to disease prevention and treatment in TCM
- **reflect on** the advantages of TCM in disease prevention and treatment

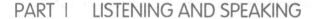

PART I   LISTENING AND SPEAKING

Before you listen

In this section you will hear a short passage entitled "Asthma and Traditional Chinese Medicine". The following words and phrases may be of help.

complication /ˌkɒmplɪˈkeɪʃ(ə)n/	n.	并发症
bronchitis /brɒŋˈkaɪtɪs/	n.	支气管炎
bronchial /ˈbrɒŋkɪəl/	a.	支气管的
sympathetic /ˌsɪmpəˈθetɪk/	a.	交感神经的
parasympathetic /ˌpærəˌsɪmpəˈθetɪk/	a.	副交感神经的
airway /ˈeəweɪ/	n.	气道
asthmatic /æsˈmætɪk/	a.	气喘的，哮喘病的
minimize /ˈmɪnɪmaɪz/	vt.	将……减到最少
constricted /kənˈstrɪktɪd/	a.	收缩的
inhaler /ɪnˈheɪlə/	n.	吸入器
mite /maɪt/	n.	螨虫
mold /məʊld/	n.	霉菌
pollen /ˈpɒlən/	n.	花粉
viral /ˈvaɪr(ə)l/	a.	病毒的
respiratory tract		呼吸道
asthmatic episode		哮喘发作

While you listen

Listen to the passage carefully and fill in each of the blanks marked from 1) to 10) according to what you have heard.

Asthma and Traditional Chinese Medicine

Asthma is said to be the most common chronic condition among children. It affects more than one child in twenty in the United States. An 1)_____ 20 million Americans suffer from asthma. Every day, 5,000 patients visit the emergency room and 14 people die due to complications of asthma.

ER-5-1
Listening
practice

Traditional Chinese medicine (TCM) has been treating asthma for thousands of years. In 1979, the World Health Organization listed forty diseases that can benefit from acupuncture. Respiratory tract diseases, including 2)_____, were included on that list. Many studies are found to relate to the success of acupuncture and Chinese herbs for the treatment of asthma in the past two decades.

Acupuncture and Chinese herbs may help improve and balance the immune system, reduce allergic reaction, adjust the 3)_____ nervous system in order to expand the walls of the airways, reduce and withdraw mucus and phlegm and increase the capacity of the lungs.

In most of the cases, acupuncture and Chinese herbs are very effective. After a series of treatments, asthmatic symptoms such as wheezing, coughing, 4)_____ and shortness of breath are reduced. The frequency of an asthmatic episode can also be minimized. In fact, many people can usually resume an active lifestyle.

However, people should always be vigilant about the serious symptoms of asthma for they can be life threatening! The airways can become so constricted that not enough oxygen can get to your 5)_____. Therefore, you should always keep a quick-relief inhaler with you at all times, even if your symptoms are under control. Please remember that asthma is about long-term management. Get 6)_____ and treatments regularly. Contact your acupuncturist about an asthma treatment plan. You should always try to keep your environment under control. Prevent 7)_____ such as household dust mites, pets, smoke, mold, pollens and 8)_____. Prevent and treat common colds and respiratory 9)_____ in their early stages. Also, watch your diet and try to avoid dairy and sugar. It is also wise to manage your 10)_____. Take action now. You could control asthma. Do not let asthma control you.

After you listen

Please discuss with your partner the following questions and give your presentation to the class.

1) How can acupuncture and Chinese herbs help patients with asthma?
2) What should patients with asthma do in their daily life to control asthma?

PART II　READING

Text A

Parkinson's Disease: Possible Treatment with Chinese Medicine

1　The characteristic symptoms of Parkinson's disease appeared in ancient Chinese medical texts that described trembling of the hands and shaking of the head. The disorder and its basis have been subjected to considerable analysis over the centuries. Syndromes in which elderly patients suffer from spontaneous shaking, or from other muscular manifestations such as paralysis or tonic spasm, are thought to be the result of yin deficiency of the kidney and liver leading to generation of "internal wind". Therefore, the therapeutic **regime** for Parkinson's disease is to nourish the kidney and liver, with focus on nourishing yin, and sedate internal wind[1]. While nourishing the kidney and liver is often accomplished by herb therapy, calming wind patterns is more frequently attempted through acupuncture therapy. In China, acupuncture and herbs have been used both independently and in combination.

Herb therapy

2　A report[2] on treatment of 40 cases of Parkinson's syndrome involved 31 male and 9 female patients, aged 54-80 years (mean 69 years), with cases classified as being severe (3 patients), moderate (27 patients), or mild (10 patients). All patients were considered to have deficiency of kidney-yin and liver-yin with stirring up of internal wind.[3] In addition, 3/4 of the patients were described as having the obstruction of phlegm in the meridians. Of the remaining 10 patients, rather than this phlegm obstruction pattern, 6 were said to have deficiency of qi and blood and 4 were said to have deficiency of yang.

3　A basic prescription was developed for treatment:

Ho-shou-wu	*Heshouwu*	何首乌	20 g
Lycium	*Gouqi*	枸杞	12 g
Cistanche	*Roucongrong*	肉苁蓉	12 g
Gastrodia	*Tianma*	天麻	15 g
Uncaria	*Gouteng*	钩藤	18 g
Cnidum	*Shechuangzi*	蛇床子	15 g
Acorus	*Changpu*	菖蒲	10 g

4　This collection of herbs, cooked to yield a decoction for drinking, would be modified

---

①　sedate internal wind: 平息内风,息风是治疗内风病证的方法。内风证主要由脏腑病变所致,其临床表现有类似风的动摇不定、急骤、变化快的特点。

②　Source: CHEN J Z, GUO J Y, SUN J, et al. TCM treatment of Parkinson's syndrome—a report of 40 cases. Journal of traditional Chinese medicine 2003, 23 (3): 168-169.

③　stirring up of internal wind: 风气内动。因其似风的急骤、动摇和多变,故名。

according to symptoms, for example:

- **Tremor**: add oyster shell (*Muli*, 牡蛎), mother of pearl (*Zhenzhumu*, 珍珠母) and **scorpion** (*Quanxie*, 全蝎).

- Rigidity:[1] add chaenomeles (*Mugua*, 木瓜), peony (*Shaoyao*, 芍药), and magnolia bark (*Houpo*, 厚朴).

- Heat pattern (constipation, aversion to heat, perspiring): add anemarrhena (*Zhimu*, 知母), phellodendron (*Huangbai*, 黄柏), gardenia (*Zhizi*, 栀子), and moutan (*Mudanpi*, 牡丹皮).

- Cold pattern (lassitude, aversion to cold, frequent urination): add eucommia (*Duzhong*, 杜仲), dipsacus (*Chuanxuduan*, 川续断), epimedium (*Yinyanghuo*, 淫羊藿), ginseng (*Renshen*, 人参), rose fruit (*Jinyingzi*, 金樱子) and alpinia (*Caodoukou*, 草豆蔻).

- Depression, anxiety, insomnia: add schizandra (*Wuweizi*, 五味子), albizzia bark (*Hehuanpi*, 合欢皮), cyperus (*Xiangfu*, 香附), and *shou wu* stem (*Shouwuteng* 首乌藤).

- For slow mental responses and **amnesia**: add polygala (*Yuanzhi*, 远志) and curcuma (*Yujin*, 郁金).

- For poor blood circulation: add salvia (*Danshen*, 丹参) and red peony (*Chishao*, 赤芍).

5 According to the authors of the report, 5 of the patients were "markedly improved" by the treatment and 15 additional cases were improved, while the remaining 10 only had slight changes. Improvement was evaluated on the basis of scores for symptoms characteristic of Parkinson's disease, including tremor, rigidity, **hypokinesis**, **gait** disturbance[2], and mask-like face[3]. They suggested that acupuncture, moxibustion, and scalp-needling might be helpful additions to the treatment.

6 Many patients with Parkinson's disease also suffer from **atherosclerosis**, and there is some thought that this problem contributes to **degeneration** of the **neurons**, perhaps as a result of insufficient blood flow or related to inflammatory processes that contribute to atherosclerosis and to neuron degeneration. In a study of patients with atherosclerosis and Parkinsonism, 60 cases were treated with the same herb formula described above, by the same research group[4]. In this case, there were 42 male and 18 female patients, aged 61-78 years (mean 67 years). In this group, it was reported that 7 of the patients were markedly improved, and 24 were improved, 15 were slightly improved, while the remaining 14 failed to respond to treatment.

---

[1] rigidity: 此处指强直,亦作"僵直"。指僵硬不能随意转动屈伸。《素问·至真要大论》:"诸躁狂越,皆属于火。诸暴强直,皆属于风。"

[2] gait disturbance: 步态障碍。帕金森病的一种特征性运动障碍,临床上存在多种表现形式,如慌张步态、冻结步态、姿势不稳致跌倒等。

[3] mask-like face: 面具脸。表情呆板,即使自己有意地做表情也显得很僵硬,好像戴了一副面具似的,医学上称为"面具脸"。

[4] Source: CHEN J Z, JIANG W, SHI J, et al. 60 cases of atherosclerotic Parkinsonism syndrome treated by supplementing liver and kidney method. Shaanxi journal of traditional Chinese medicine 1999, 20 (1): 19.

7　In another study[①] of Chinese herbal medicine, 700 cases of treatments of Parkinson's patients at a hospital were reviewed; 50 of them, involving prolonged therapy, were analyzed. The case reports were concerning 32 men and 18 women, with age ranging from 35 to 75 years. The patients were divided into three categories by the traditional method of differentiation and were treated with herbs accordingly. Because these were case studies, rather than a specific prescription, commonly used herbs were mentioned.

- For yin deficiency of the kidney and liver, the main herbs were: rehmannia (raw and processed *Dihuang* 生地黄和熟地黄), ho-shou-wu (*Heshouwu*, 何首乌), cornus (*Shanzhuyu*, 山茱萸), tortoise shell (*Guijia*, 龟甲), scrophularia (*Xuanshen*, 玄参).

- For qi stagnation and blood stasis type, the main herbs were: salvia (*Danshen*, 丹参), red peony (*Chishao*, 赤芍), carthamus (*Honghua*, 红花), persica (*Taoren*, 桃仁), cnidium (*Shechuangzi*, 蛇床子), achyranthes (*Niuxi*, 牛膝), tang-kuei (*Danggui*, 当归), eupolyphaga (*Dibiechong*, 地鳖虫), and pangolin scale (*Chuanshanjia*, 穿山甲).

- For deficiency of qi and blood, the main herbs were: ginseng (*Renshen*, 人参), astragalus (*Huangqi*, 黄芪), atractylodes (*Cangzhu*, 苍术), tang-kuei (*Danggui*, 当归), rehmannia (*Dihuang*, 地黄), licorice (*Gancao*, 甘草), peony (*Shaoyao*, 芍药), salvia (*Danshen*, 丹参), schizandra (*Wuweizi*, 五味子), and ligustrum (*Nüzhenzi*, 女贞子).

8　The formulas would be modified according to specific symptoms, for example, to address continuous trembling, use **antelope** horn (*Lingyangjiao*, 羚羊角)[②], uncaria (*Gouteng*, 钩藤), and gastrodia (*Tianma*, 天麻); additional wind-sedating substances might also be used.

9　The herbs were prepared in the form of decoction, which was given in two doses per day. Most of the patients took the decoctions daily for three months. Many of the patients were taking standard Western medicines at the start of the treatment and, according to the authors, several were able to reduce their dosage or discontinue these medicines during or after treatment with the decoctions. The authors reported that of the 50 patients analyzed, the treatment was markedly effective in 15 cases, and somewhat effective in 24 cases, the remainder (11 cases) did not respond to therapy significantly.

Acupuncture therapy

10　In a study[③] of acupuncture therapy **administered** to 29 patients with Parkinson's disease, the patients were treated every other day for three months. Western drugs (mainly l-dopa[④], **dopaminergic receptor** stimulants, and **anticholinergics**) were used as per usual practice; a control group taking Western drugs alone (24 patients) was also **monitored.**

11　Two sets of acupuncture points served as the basis of therapy, and they were

①　Source: LI G H. Clinical observation on Parkinson's disease treated by integration of traditional Chinese and Western medicine. Journal of traditional Chinese medicine 1995, 15 (3): 163-169.

②　antelope horn: 羚羊角，中药名。本品为雄性牛科动物赛加羚羊 (Saiga tataricaLinnaeus) 的角。赛加羚羊被列入《世界自然保护联盟》(IUCN) 2012 年濒危物种红色名录 ver3.1— 极危 (CR)，严禁狩猎。

③　Source: ZHUANG X L, WANG L L, ZHOU Y S. Acupuncture treatment of Parkinson's disease—a report of 29 cases. Journal of traditional Chinese medicine, 2000, 20 (4): 263-267.

④　L-dopa: Levodopa 左旋多巴，又名左多巴，为抗震颤麻痹药。

administered alternately: Group1: *Sishencong* (EX-HN1), *Quchi* (LI11), *Waiguan* (TE5), *Yanglingquan* (GB34), *Zusanli* (ST36), and *Fenglong* (ST40).

Group 2: *Benshen* (GB13), *Fengchi* (GB20), *Baihui* (GV20), *Hegu* (LI4), *Sanyinjiao* (SP6), and *Taichong* (LR3).

12　Electrostimulation was administered to *Sishencong* (EX-HN1), *Benshen* (GB13), and *Fengchi* (GB20) for 15 minutes, using a frequency of 180 cycles/minute, with the **intensity** adjusted to the tolerance limit for the patient. To avoid reduction of sensitivity to the **stimulus** over the course of the treatment, a continuous wave[①] was used initially, but then followed by a "disperse-dense" wave[②]. The other points were needled with the conventional manual method of stimulation. Needle retention was 40 minutes. Additional acupuncture points would be used for treating specific symptoms, so that, with most points being **bilateral**, about 12-16 needles were used in each treatment.

13　A follow-up study[③] was conducted by the same group, focusing on the *Sishencong* (EX-HN1) points with a comparison group treated with four points on the limbs (arms and legs). According to the report, acupuncture increased the **cerebral** blood flow **velocity**, which was taken as a sign of improved circulation to the affected parts of the brain, and the *Sishencong* (EX-HN1) points had a more notable effect on the brain circulation.

14　Another report[④] on acupuncture also focused on acupuncture near the scalp point *Baihui* (GV20). In this case, acupuncture was performed along the scalp from *Qianding* (GV21) to *Baihui* (GV20), using the standard techniques of scalp acupuncture. In addition to the scalp points, *Yamen* (GV15), *Fengchi* (GB20), and other points at the neck would be treated by standard acupuncture.

15　It was noted that there were some responses immediately after treatment, with calming of tremor in 2/3 of the patients. Among 24 patients that completed three months of therapy, 6 were said to show marked improvement, and the other 18 moderately effective (there were 43 patients starting the therapy, and some discontinued due to lack of efficacy).

Summary

16　Both acupuncture and herb therapies have been reported to show benefits for some patients suffering from Parkinson's disease. The herb therapies are mainly high dosage preparations of herbs that nourish yin and blood, sedate wind, **vitalize** blood circulation, and resolve phlegm-obstruction of the meridians. Acupuncture is administered every other day, usually with prolonged stimulus (30-40 minutes). Prompt effects of acupuncture (right after treatment) may be observed, but standard therapeutic regimens are three months.

---

① continuous wave: 连续波, 为电针刺激参数。

② "disperse-dense" wave: 疏密波, 为电针输出波形之一。

③ Source: WANG L L, HE C, ZHAO M, et al. Influence of acupuncture on brain blood flowing state in Parkinson's patients. Chinese acupuncture and moxibustion, 1999, (2): 115-116.

④ Source: XI G F, CAI D H, CHEN G M, et al. Impact of electrostimulation at scalp points on tremor-myeloectropotential in Parkinson's disease patients. Shanghai journal of acupuncture and moxibustion, 1996, 15 (3): 5-6.

Reference: DHARMANANDA S. Parkinson's disease: possible treatment with Chinese medicine [EB/OL]. [2022-11-03]. http://www.itmonline.org/arts/parkinsons.htm.

New words

regime /reɪˈʒiːm/	*n.*	a method or system of organizing or managing sth. 方法
tremor /ˈtremə/	*n.*	an involuntary quivering movement 震颤
scorpion /ˈskɔːpɪən/	*n.*	a small creature like an insect with eight legs, two front claws (curved and pointed arms) and a long tail that curves over its back and can give a poisonous sting 蝎子
amnesia /æmˈniːzɪə/	*n.*	a partial or total loss of memory 健忘症
hypokinesis /ˌhaɪpəʊkɪˈniːsɪs/	*n.*	decreased bodily movement 运动减退
gait /geɪt/	*n.*	a person's manner of walking 步态
atherosclerosis /ˌæθərəʊsklɪəˈrəʊsɪs/	*n.*	a disease of the arteries characterized by the deposition of fatty material on their inner walls 动脉粥样硬化
degeneration /dɪˌdʒenəˈreɪʃ(ə)n/	*n.*	deterioration and loss of function in the cells of a tissue or organ 退化，恶化
neuron /ˈnjʊərɒn/	*n.*	a specialized cell transmitting nerve impulses; a nerve cell 神经元
antelope /ˈæntɪləʊp/	*n.*	a swift-running deer-like ruminant (反刍动物) with smooth hair and upward-pointing horns 羚羊
administer /ədˈmɪnɪstə/	*vt*	dispense or apply (a remedy or drug) 给予 (药物)
dopaminergic /ˌdəʊpəmɪˈnɜːdʒɪk/	*a.*	releasing or involving dopamine as a neurotransmitter 多巴胺能的
receptor /rɪˈseptə/	*n.*	an organ or cell able to respond to light, heat, or other external stimulus and transmit a signal to a sensory nerve 受体
anticholinergics /ˌæntɪˌkəʊlɪˈnɜːdʒɪks/	*n.*	an anticholinergic drug 抗胆碱能药物
monitor /ˈmɒnɪtə/	*vt.*	observe and check the progress or quality of (sth.) over a period of time 监控
intensity /ɪnˈtensɪti/	*n.*	the quality of being intense 强度
stimulus /ˈstɪmjʊləs/	*n.*	a thing or event that evokes a specific functional reaction in an organ or tissue 刺激物

bilateral /baɪˈlæt(ə)r(ə)l/	*a.*	having or relating to two sides 两侧的
cerebral /ˈserɪbr(ə)l/	*a.*	relating to the brain 大脑的
velocity /vɪˈlɒsɪti/	*n.*	the speed of sth. in a given direction 速率，速度
vitalize /ˈvaɪt(ə)laɪz/	*vt.*	give strength and energy to 激发

Phrases and expressions

tonic spasm	强直性痉挛
internal wind	内风
therapeutic regime for Parkinson's disease	帕金森病的治疗方案
phlegm obstruction	痰阻
frequent urination	尿频
inflammatory process	炎性过程
neuron degeneration	神经元变性
dopaminergic receptor stimulant	多巴胺受体兴奋剂
as per usual practice	照例
tolerance limit	耐受限度
needle retention	留针
follow-up study	随访研究
blood flow velocity	血流速度

Task One　Preview

1. Learn the following roots and affixes. Write out the Chinese meaning of the given words.

Roots/ Affixes	Meaning of roots/affixes	Words	Chinese meaning of the given words
-al	pertaining to	cerebral	_____
		colossal	_____
athero	of or pertaining to arteriosclerosis	atherogenesis	_____
		atherosclerosis	_____
-atric	treat, medical healing	bariatric	_____
		pediatric	_____
cept	take	accept	_____
		receptor	_____
chol	gallbladder	cholesterol	_____
		cholinergic	_____
-ence	action, process	absence	_____
		adolescence	_____

gen-	line of descent	genetics	_____
		genocide	_____
homo-	same	homogeneous	_____
		homosexual	_____
-itude	quality or state	attitude	_____
		lassitude	_____
kine	movement	kinesthesia	_____
		kinesiology	_____
-lysis	breakdown, destruction	hemolysis	_____
		paralysis	_____
matur	ripe	immaturity	_____
		maturate	_____
-mne	memory	amnesia	_____
		automnesia	_____
neur (o)	nerve	neuroma	_____
		neuron	_____
-rrhea	flow, flowing	agalorrhea	_____
		diarrhea	_____
sta-	stay, stand still	stagnate	_____
		stasis	_____
veloc (i)	speed, swift, rapid	velocity	_____
		velocimetry	_____
vita	life, living	vitalism	_____
		vitamin	_____

2. Write down the questions you would like to ask or discuss about the text.

_____

_____

_____

Task Two   Speaking

1. Answer the following questions according to the text.

1) What is the TCM therapeutic principle for Parkinson's disease?

2) If a Parkinson's patient has a dull reaction, what kinds of herbs should be added to the basic prescription?

3) What are the characteristic symptoms of Parkinson's disease?

4) Why do many Parkinson's patients also suffer from atherosclerosis?

5) What are the main herbs for Parkinson's patients with yin deficiency of the kidney and liver?

6) Why are both a continuous wave and a "disperse-dense" wave used over the course of acupuncture treatment for Parkinson's patients?

7) What can acupuncture do to the affected parts of the brain?

8) What are the benefits of herb therapies for some patients suffering from Parkinson's disease?

2. Work in pairs or groups and exchange views on the following news.

Hong Kong Allows Hospitals to Try Chinese Herbs for SARS

HONG KONG—Desperately searching for a cure for SARS, Hong Kong's hospitals will allow the use of TCM for the first time since World War II, the city's health authority said on Monday.

The surprise move came after Hong Kong announced another six deaths from severe acute respiratory syndrome (SARS), and as more physicians and nurses in the territory began taking Chinese herbs to protect themselves against the disease. "We are open to the use of Chinese medicine," said Liu Shao-haei, senior executive manager of the Hospital Authority. "But we will see if the patient wants it, how it is to be applied and if the patient's condition allows for such alternative types of treatment," he told a news conference.

Hospitals in the city have not used TCM for treatment since the Japanese occupation in the early 1940s. But the medicines, mostly derived plants, are extremely popular in the city of seven million. Since the outbreak of SARS in February, hundreds of thousands of people are using traditional recipes to ward off the disease.

Some physicians and relatives of patients in Hong Kong have been lobbying for the use of Chinese herbs to treat SARS, especially after officials recently said a cocktail of the anti-viral drug, ribavirin (利巴韦林), and steroids (类固醇) was not working for a small but growing number of patients.

A team of Chinese medicine experts at Hong Kong's Chinese University put together a recipe in mid-April as part of an urgent effort to bring down the rate of infection among front-line medical staff.

Front-line health care workers are especially vulnerable to SARS and up to a quarter of people infected in Hong Kong are doctors and nurses who had attended to severely ill SARS patients. "Chinese medicine is most suitable for prevention of the illness and for treatment in the initial and middle stages of the illness," Dr. Cen Ze-bo, from the School of Chinese Medicine at the Chinese University, said.

Health care workers at the Prince of Wales Hospital, site of Hong Kong's first SARS outbreak, have been taking herbs in a granulated form, since mid-April. The granules are dissolved in hot water and the mixture is then consumed once or twice daily. Some of its main ingredients are wild barley (coix) and *Banlangen* (isatis root), a dried plant root. Cen said the recipe was similar to those used in hospitals in China's southern province of Guangdong, where the disease emerged in November.

"We will need maybe a month to see how effective it is in controlling the infection rate among hospital staff," he said. Hospitals in Guangdong are using a mixture of both

Western and Chinese medicine to fight the epidemic, Cen noted.

Topic for discussion: What do you think of the role of TCM in the prevention and treatment of epidemic diseases?

Task Three　Vocabulary

1. Match up each word in Column A with its appropriate definition from Column B.

Column A

1) cerebral

2) amnesia

3) lassitude

4) rigidity

5) efficacy

6) atherosclerosis

7) degeneration

8) electrostimulation

9) decoction

10) hypokinesis

11) paralysis

12) phlegm

Column B

a. the quality or state of stiffness or inflexibility

b. diminished or abnormally slow movement

c. partial or total loss of memory

d. a liquid medicine made from an extract of water-soluble substances

e. complete loss of strength in an affected limb or muscle group

f. of or relating to the brain or cerebrum

g. electric stimulation of a nerve, muscle, etc.

h. the quality of being successful in producing an intended result

i. a state or feeling of weariness, diminished energy, or listlessness

j. a disease of the arteries caused by buildup of fatty deposits

k. thick, slimy liquid brought up from the throat by coughing

l. the process of declining from a higher to a lower level of effective power or vitality or essential quality

2. Fill in the blanks with the words given below. Change the form where necessary.

account	unresponsive	resolution	suppress	susceptible
massive	diagnose	highlight	solve	phenomenon
immature	inaccessible	common	adult	facilitate

Treating Children with Traditional Chinese Medicine

Pediatrics is one of the oldest specialties within traditional Chinese medicine (TCM) and dates from the early first millennium. Since that time, there has been continuous development in the 1) ＿＿＿＿＿＿ and treatment of children's diseases. Past generations of Chinese doctors have discovered various characteristics that are 2) ＿＿＿＿＿＿ in all children. The various modalities of TCM have been providing children with 3) ＿＿＿＿＿＿ to their health problems for more than 2,000 years.

TCM is a noninvasive healing modality that 4) ＿＿＿＿＿＿ the body's natural ability to heal itself by restoring harmony and balance to the entire individual. According to TCM, children are not just considered miniature 5) ＿＿＿＿＿＿. They are believed to be immature both physically and functionally; most common pediatric complaints are due to this 6) ＿＿＿＿＿＿. TCM states that because children's bodies are immature and therefore inherently weak, they are 7) _____ to diseases that affect the lungs such as colds, coughs, allergies and asthma and the spleen (or digestive complaints) such as colic, vomiting, diarrhea, indigestion, and stomach aches.

TCM has been shown to offer substantial clinical benefits to patients who have been 8) _____ to other forms of treatment. The treatment of these diseases using TCM have less side effects and are curative, as they aim to eliminate the pathology of the disease instead of controlling or 9) _____ the symptoms. In most chronic diseases, Western medicine takes a more reactive approach to medicine, in that the symptoms are treated. In TCM a proactive approach is taken, in that the whole body and how it functions is taken into 10) _____ .

Task Four　Translation

1. Study the following sentences and pay attention to the underlined parts.

1) The disorder and its basis have been subjected to considerable analysis over the centuries. (para. 1)

2) In China, acupuncture and herbs have been used both independently and in combination. (para. 1)

3) Improvement was evaluated on the basis of scores for symptoms characteristic of Parkinson's disease, including tremor, rigidity, hypokinesis, gait disturbance, and mask-like face. (para. 5)

4) The case reports were concerning 32 men and 18 women, with age ranging from 35 to 75 years. (para. 7)

5) In a study of acupuncture therapy administered to 29 patients with Parkinson's disease, the patients were treated every other day for three months. (para. 10)

6) It was noted that there were some responses immediately after treatment, with calming of tremor in 2/3 of the patients. (para. 15)

2. Translate the following sentences into English.

1) 本文主题是肝癌患者一线治疗的临床疗效。

2) 某些药物如果与某些食物、酒或其他药物一起服用,正常剂量下也可能会产生毒性。

3) 这项研究最吸引人的发现是:即使排除了哮喘或目前的吸烟人群,该人群中发生心衰的比率也很高。

4) 针灸可以治疗一系列疾病,包括妇科疾病、泌尿系统疾病、精神压力和背痛。

5) 作者提出了使用止痛剂(analgesics)和镇静剂(sedatives)治疗车祸中受伤患者的方法。

6) 值得注意的是,这种延迟有可能会增加手术难度,降低总体改善程度。

Text B

Childhood Asthma: The Traditional Chinese Medicine Approach

1   Asthma is the most common chronic disease of childhood. Improperly treated asthma may lead to a lifetime of asthma. Children can sometimes outgrow their asthma and half of these children will see a lessening of their symptoms as they move into adolescence. However, approximately 50% of this group will see their asthma return, often when they are in their 30s and 40s. Asthma can cause death and approximately 10 children and 450 adults die from asthma each year in Canada.

2   Fifty-two percent of children currently receiving treatment from a modern medical doctor have poorly controlled asthma, yet 88% of parents continue to believe their child's asthma is controlled.

3   Traditional Chinese medicine (TCM) prides itself on its ability to treat and assess each person as an individual, not based entirely on a disease (i.e., asthma) or symptoms (i.e., cough, wheezing etc.). In this ancient form of medicine, healing is based on the restoration of harmony and balance within the body. This balance is restored through the use of Chinese herbal medicine, acupuncture, dietary therapy, exercise (physical and mental) and tuina (Chinese massage).

4   Asthma is discussed under the TCM disease categories of "cough" and "**panting and wheezing**". The basis of the modern TCM approach to treatment of asthma was first discussed in detail by a famous doctor named Zhu Danxi[①] (600 years ago). Since then the treatment of this disease has been refined and improved upon by many generations of Chinese doctors.

Causes of asthma in kids

5   In TCM, the five causes of all illnesses (including asthma) are improper diet, emotions, lifestyle, external environment and constitution (i.e., **genetics**). Any or all of these factors may **aggravate** or cause asthma. Similar to adult asthma, **pediatric** asthma is characterized by two stages: acute and **remission**. Triggers for acute attacks in children include **allergens** (i.e., external environment), environmental **exposures** (i.e., lifestyle), infections, and strong emotions (not common in children). Studies have shown children with a family history of asthma are more likely to develop it. In addition, most children with asthma (up to 80%) also suffer from significant allergies including higher **incidences** of allergic **rhinitis** and eczema. A child with a weaker constitution, such as a child whose mother smoked while pregnant or a child born with a lower birth weight, are also more likely to suffer from asthma.

6   TCM recognizes that children have unique physiological characteristics and cannot be

---

① Zhu Danxi: 朱丹溪,元代著名医学家。

considered as just **miniature** adults. When treating asthma, one of the main differences of pediatric physiology is that a child's digestion is immature, especially before the age of six years old when most asthma begins. This immaturity and weakness of the digestion (spleen) **predisposes** a child to experience an incomplete breakdown of food and the accumulation of phlegm. It is said in TCM that, "the spleen is the source of phlegm production" and "the lungs are the place where phlegm is stored".

Acute and chronic stages of pediatric asthma

7   Chinese medicine divides asthma into two stages—acute and chronic. Both types share the main symptoms of asthma, which include shortness of breath, tightness in the chest, coughing and wheezing. Due to a child's pure yang constitution,[①] the hot type of asthma is much more common.

8   The "hot type" will present with some or all of the following symptoms: cough with yellow phlegm, fever, red face, yellowish urine, dry **stools** or constipation, thirst with a desire to drink, red tongue with a yellow coating[②] and a slippery rapid pulse.

9   The "cold type" is really a pattern of acute asthma without heat and may include the following symptoms: cough with clear, watery, white-colored phlegm, a cold body with no perspiration, dull and lusterless complexion, cold limbs, no thirst or only thirst for hot drinks, thin white or slimy tongue coating, and a superficial, slippery pulse.

10   In general, the acute stage or asthma attacks should be treated with modern medicine (one or two days) in conjunction with TCM. Most children under a doctor's care will already be taking some form of **inhaled broncho-dilating** medication, which can be convenient and practical.

11   TCM is also effective during these acute **episodes** and the most important modality used in the treatment of pediatric asthma is Chinese herbal medicine. The herbal formulas used are **customized** according to the child's TCM pattern, presenting symptoms and the stage of the patient's asthma. The formula usually consists of around 10 to 15 **ingredients**, chosen based on the individual's clinical presentation. At this stage, the child is closely monitored with clinical visits occurring every four to seven days. Upon return visits, the formula is modified as the patient's condition improves. Acupuncture can also be helpful in the acute stage and moxibustion may be more useful in the chronic stage.

12   In the remission stage, some of the above symptoms have now been eliminated and reduced in severity. However, the clinical presentation is now one of deficiency rather than excess; the child presents with signs of qi deficiency and deep-lying phlegm during the remission stage. Symptoms of qi deficiency may include a pale complexion, fatigue, lack of strength, spontaneous perspiration, cold limbs, decreased appetite, cough with phlegm, incomplete or loose stools, **bedwetting**, shortness of breath (especially on **exertion**), pale tongue and/or a weak pulse. Indicators that phlegm is present include a cough with copious

---

①   pure yang constitution: 纯阳体质，为小儿生理、病理特点之一。
②   coating: 此处指舌苔。

white watery phlegm, nasal obstruction, a clear **runny** nose, and a **slimy** tongue fur.

13   During the remission stage, the focus of treatment is on preventing acute attacks through strengthening the body. Once again, the main treatment is herbal medicine; however, the nature of the ingredients is now much different. The medicinals work to supplement and **fortify** the body's qi in order to strengthen the body's defensive qi (or immunity). The main organs that need to be strengthened in pediatric asthma are the spleen and lungs. In adults, the treatment during the remission stage may also include supplementation of the kidneys. In conjunction with these medicinals, the TCM doctor also prescribes ingredients to transform the remaining or deep-lying phlegm in the body.

14   In order to prevent an acute attack and strengthen the body, proper diet and exercise are also very important during this stage. In addition, other methods of treatment may be used. One such treatment is "winter tonification" which is a paste form of herbal medicine that is taken for six weeks in the winter to prevent the attack of the common cold and asthma for the entire year. Another **adjunct** modality to the interior administration of Chinese herbs is herbal plasters that are applied to acupuncture points on the child's back. This treatment is done once a week for three weeks in the winter and repeated in the summer for three weeks.

Prognosis of treatment

15   With persistent treatment and by modifying the herbal formula according to the patient's clinical presentation even some of the most severe forms of pediatric asthma can be cured (i.e., three years without an exacerbation) using TCM. If a cure cannot be achieved, the child's asthma will at least be better controlled with a decrease in daytime and nighttime symptoms. In general, the longer a person suffers from a disease such as asthma, the more difficult it will be to treat. Moreover, the TCM treatment results of asthma are best if the child has not yet reached **puberty**.

Reference: HELMER R. Childhood asthma: the TCM approach [EB/OL]. (2004-05-15) [2015-11-09] http://vitalitymagazine.com/article/childhood-asthma/.

New words

pant /pænt/	vi.	breathe with short, quick breaths, typically from exertion or excitement 喘息
genetics /dʒəˈnetɪks/	n.	the qualities and characteristics passed from each generation of living things to the next 遗传,遗传特征
aggravate /ˈæɡrəveɪt/	vt.	make an illness or a bad or unpleasant situation worse 加重,使恶化
pediatric /piːdɪˈætrɪk/	a.	relating to the branch of medicine dealing with children and their diseases 儿科的
remission /rɪˈmɪʃ(ə)n/	n.	a temporary diminution of the severity of disease or pain 减轻,缓和

笔记

allergen /ˈæləstdʒ(ə)n/	*n.*	a substance that causes an allergy 过敏原
exposure /ɪkˈspəʊʒə/	*n.*	the state of having no protection from contact with sth. harmful 暴露
incidence /ˈɪnsɪd(ə)ns/	*n.*	the occurrence, rate, or frequency of a disease, crime, or other undesirable thing 发生率
rhinitis /raɪˈnaɪtɪs/	*n.*	a condition in which the inside of the nose becomes swollen and sore, caused by an infection or an allergy 鼻炎
miniature /ˈmɪnɪtʃə/	*a.*	very small of its kind 微小的，微型的
predispose /ˌpriːdɪˈspəʊz/	*vt.*	make it likely that you will suffer from a particular illness 使易患病
stool /stuːl/	*n.*	a piece of solid waste from your body 粪便
inhale /ɪnˈheɪl/	*vt.*	breathe in 吸入
broncho-dilating /ˈbrɒŋkəʊ daɪˈleɪtɪŋ/	*a.*	related to the dilation of the bronchial tubes 扩张支气管的
episode /ˈepɪsəʊd/	*n.*	a finite period in which sb. is affected by a specified illness（某疾病）的发作期
customize /ˈkʌstəmaɪz/	*vt.*	modify (sth.) to suit a particular individual or task 定制
ingredient /ɪnˈgriːdɪənt/	*n.*	one of the things from which sth. is made 成分，组成部分
bedwetting /ˈbedwetɪŋ/	*n.*	involuntary urination during the night 尿床
exertion /ɪgˈzəːʃn/	*n.*	physical or mental effort 努力，费力
runny /ˈrʌnɪ/	*a.*	(of a person's nose) producing or discharging mucus; running（鼻）流涕的
slimy /ˈslaɪmɪ/	*a.*	covered by or resembling slime 黏滑的
fortify /ˈfɔːtɪfaɪ/	*n.*	strengthen 增强
adjunct /ˈædʒʌŋ(k)t/	*vt.* *a.*	connected or added to sth., typically in an auxiliary way 附属的，辅助的
prognosis /prɒgˈnəʊsɪs/	*n.*	a forecast of the likely outcome of a situation 预测；[医] 预后
puberty /ˈpjuːbəti/	*n.*	the period during which adolescents reach sexual maturity and become capable of reproduction 青春期

笔记

120

Phrases and expressions

pride ... on	对……感到自豪
pediatric asthma	小儿哮喘
environmental exposure	环境暴露（接触）
higher incidences of allergic rhinitis	过敏性鼻炎发生率较高
miniature adult	成人的微缩版
accumulation of phlegm	痰积
tightness in the chest	胸闷
slippery rapid pulse	脉象滑数
lusterless complexion	面色无华
in conjunction with	与……协力
broncho-dilating medication	支气管扩张药
acute episode	急性发作
clinical presentation	临床表现
deep-lying phlegm	伏痰
remission stage	缓解期
decreased appetite	食欲下降
copious white watery phlegm	大量的白稀痰
acute attack	急性发作

Task One Preview

1. Learn the following roots and affixes. Write out the Chinese meaning of the given words.

Roots/ Affixes	Meaning of roots/affixes	Words	Chinese Meaning of the given words
bronch (o)	windpipe	bronchospasm	_____
		bronchus	_____
-en	cause to be	worsen	_____
		lessen	_____
exter-	outside	exterior	_____
		externalize	_____
forti	strong	fortification	_____
		fortify	_____
-gnosis	knowledge	diagnosis	_____
		prognosis	_____
grav	heavy	aggravate	_____
		gravid	_____

hal	breath, breathe	exhale	_____
		inhale	_____
-ic	of	alcoholic	_____
		allergic	_____
im-	no, not	immoral	_____
		impassable	_____
-ity	condition or quality of being...	immaturity	_____
		parity	_____
junct	join	adjunct	_____
		junction	_____
-ment	the act or state or fact of...	equipment	_____
		treatment	_____
mini-	minor	miniature	_____
		minimum	_____
out-	beyond, more than	outgrow	_____
		outlook	_____
ped	child	misopedy	_____
		pediatric	_____
rhin (o)	nose	arhinia	_____
		rhinitis	_____
super-	above, over	superficial	_____
		supervision	_____
- (i)um	denoting singular grammatical number	bacterium	_____
		millennium	_____

2. Write down the questions you would like to ask or discuss about the text.

_____

_____

_____

Task Two   Vocabulary

Choose the word or phrase that can best complete the statements.

1) According to the authors, the clinical _____ of sarcoidosis (肉状瘤病) is varied and nonspecific and the diagnosis is easily mistaken.

   A. presentation   B. result   C. treatment   D. observation

2) Four in every 1,000 children aged 6 to 12 in China have autism, a (n) _____ that experts say is higher than expected.

   A. number   B. rate   C. incidence   D. percentage

3) Some experts are carrying out a study to determine whether depressed mood or life

events will _____ inflammatory bowel disease.

    A. stimulate   B. exacerbate   C. treat   D. promote

4) This review is the first to attempt identification of studies investigating life expectancy in hereditary diseases which _____ to early-onset tumors.

    A. predispose   B. lead   C. relate   D. result

5) Phlegm-dampness, dampness-heat and qi-deficiency _____ were the three dominant constitutional types seen in the metabolic syndrome patients.

    A. situations   B. conditions   C. circumstances   D. constitutions

6) Recovery is ascribed after at least 4 months following the onset of _____, during which a relapse has not occurred.

    A. treatment   B. cure   C. remission   D. operation

7) Learning disabilities are not _____ and thus adults with learning disabilities need to learn practical strategies.

    A. cured   B. found   C. discovered   D. outgrown

8) In recent years, significant amounts of studies have shown that TCM and its active _____ have obvious hypoglycemic effect (降糖效果).

    A. activity   B. performance   C. ingredients   D. parts

9) *Shenling Baizhu* Powder is an amazing mixture of both herbs that can be used long-term because of their slow _____ of digestive process, but it also includes some quick acting ingredients as well.

    A. tonification   B. stimulation   C. motion   D. inspiration

10) The purpose of this study was to measure the brain temperature of human volunteers _____ intranasal cooling using non-invasive magnetic resonance imaging (MRI) methods.

    A. subjected by   B. subjecting to   C. subjected to   D. subject with

11) According to TCM, if the Heart Meridian is _____ by phlegm, dementia and loss of consciousness may occur.

    A. destruct   B. instructed   C. constructed   D. obstructed

12) Age-related macular (黄斑的) _____ is the commonest cause of severe loss of central vision in people aged over 50 in the Western world.

    A. regression   B. degeneration   C. generation   D. regeneration

13) Trained members of the public will be able to supply and _____ emergency "rescue" medicines to individuals in emergency circumstances.

    A. distribute   B. provide   C. manage   D. administer

14) Almost 14% patients defined as particularly _____ to adverse drug events were prescribed one or more high risk drugs.

    A. relevant   B. vulnerable   C. related   D. responsive

15) Despite growing recognition of the problem, the obesity _____ continues in the U.S., and obesity rates are increasing around the world.

    A. epidemic   B. situation   C. phenomenon   D. condition

Task Three　Translation

Translate the following expressions into English.

1) 治未病
2) 急者缓之
3) 既病防变
4) 未病先防
5) 留者攻之
6) 劳者温之
7) 宣肺止咳平喘
8) 攻补兼施
9) 补中益气
10) 理气解郁
11) 疏肝解郁
12) 活血化瘀
13) 养心安神
14) 暴怒伤阴,暴喜伤阳
15) 喜怒不节则伤脏
16) 配伍禁忌
17) 膏药疗法
18) 贴敷疗法
19) 舒筋活络
20) 春夏养阳,秋冬养阴

PART Ⅲ   TRANSLATION AND WRITING

How to Make Suggestions from a Traditional Chinese Medicine Perspective

Today more and more people, not only Chinese but also foreigners, are discovering traditional Chinese medicine (TCM) as safe, effective alternatives for the prevention and treatment of diseases. However, many of them know little about TCM. They demand effective suggestions under some circumstances. To make suggestions, one should 1) introduce some related information（介绍相关信息）; 2) use formulas of making suggestions（使用建议惯用语）; 3) make suggestions in an orderly way（列举建议）; 4) provide references to add validity to your argument（提供建议理由）; and 5) express your wishes（表达祝愿）.

The following sentences or expressions are commonly used to make suggestions.

1) To let go of things that are painful or harmful is important to both our emotional and physical well-being.

摒弃痛苦的、有害的事情有益于身心健康。

2) So, my advice to you is this. Acknowledge how you are feeling. It is common for people to avoid feeling emotions that are overwhelming and/or unpleasant, but it is only in acknowledging our feelings that we may begin to deal with them and move on.

因此，我给你的建议就是：承认你的感受。人们常常回避强烈的以及/或者不愉快的情感，但是只有承认，才有可能着手解决，继续前行。

3) When you are speaking with your acupuncturist, be honest. Tell them how you are feeling.

与针灸师沟通时要实事求是，告诉他们你的感受。

4) If you have emotional issues that you are having difficulty dealing with, I urge you to try these exercises and foods, and if they are not enough, to seek out an acupuncturist and work with them to deal with the issues once and for all.

如果有难以解决的情感问题，我劝你尝试这些运动和食物。如果还是不行，就寻求针灸师的帮助，一起彻底解决这些问题。

5）Another thing that you can do to help with grief is to massage along the Lung Meridian, which is located on the arms.

另一个有助于消除悲伤的方法就是按摩位于手臂的肺经。

6) The ancient classics suggest that one should go by the laws of yin and yang, do body-building exercises best suited to one's conditions, practice temperance in food and drink, follow a regular schedule in daily life, and keep calm and cheerful.

古代典籍建议要遵循阴阳之道，根据自身条件合理运动、节制饮食、生活规律、保持平静愉悦的心态。

7）The ancient classics proposes regulating the emotions by keeping the heart calm and cheerful and the mind free of worries.

古代典籍主张保持平和、愉快和无忧无虑的心态以调节情志。

8) When one is in a bad or abnormal mood, one should try to adjust and control it lest it go to an extreme.

情绪不佳或异常时,要努力调节、控制,防止其过激。

9) Timely adjustment of one's emotions with a view to preventing them from going to the extreme is an effective method of disease prevention.

及时调整情绪、防止情绪过激是预防疾病的有效方法。

10) When faced with something exasperating, one should calmly consider which is more important—anger or health?

面对令人气恼的事情时,应该冷静地思考哪一个更重要:愤怒还是健康？

11) When in great distress or depression, one may listen to a favorite piece of music or when one is in great sorrow following some misfortune, one may stay with relatives or good friends for a period of time

特别悲痛或抑郁时,可以听喜欢的音乐;灾难后无比悲伤时,可以和亲戚或好友在一起待一段时间。

12) One should respond promptly and effectively to emotional distress and should cultivate habits and thought patterns that help one avoid frequent experience of emotional excess.

应该及时有效地应对情感抑郁,应该养成避免经常发生过激情绪的习惯和思维方式。

13) Since excessive emotions arise because of derangements in the functions of the internal organs and disorders of the circulation of qi and blood, one can deal with the effects of the emotions by making efforts to correct these internal imbalances.

脏腑功能紊乱、气血循环失调会导致情志过极,可以通过努力纠正内部的不平衡来调节情志。

14) Aside from receiving acupuncture and herbs from practitioners, the individual is expected to regulate daily life.

除了接受医生的针灸和中药治疗外,个人也要进行日常生活调整。

15) Since excessive emotions lead to diseases, one must cultivate a mental condition that is calm.

过激的情绪会致病,因此必须养成平和的精神状态。

Sample

Laughter and Joy—The Best Medicine

People always go to see a doctor when they are ill. They seldom realize that their trouble may be caused by emotions. According to traditional Chinese medicine (TCM), emotional injuries are a major cause of disease. Over 2,000 years ago, *Huangdi's Inner of Cannon of Medicine*, China's first substantial medical work, said, "Five emotions come from the five internal organs—joy, anger, grief, excess thinking and fear. Joy hurts the heart, anger hurts the liver, excess thinking hurts the spleen, grief hurts the lung and fear hurts the kidney." 1) What this meant is that emotional factors are natural human states, but that an excess of any of them can cause diseases.

2) Chinese researchers on disease prevention attach great importance to the functions of the emotions in keeping physically fit and healthy. They theorize an interaction between the emotions and the body, believing that a good emotional state can help improve general well-being and increase longevity. They put much emphasis on a peaceful state of mind and broadmindedness.

But how can we keep a positive state of mind? Here are some suggestions for achieving that goal. 3) Develop a strong sense of morality, an ethical code and live by it. Unselfish and noble-spirited people are broadminded, optimistic and always in high spirits. Jealousy, envy, hate and anxiety are negative states that rebound on those who indulge in them. Try to see the "broad picture" in life. Don't worry about trifles and don't be overly critical. 4) It is well known that some people fall into a depression after retirement, while those who keep active and have a cause or activity tend to be better off emotionally and physically.

5) For good health and longevity, you should learn to control your emotions, develop a carefree, relaxed lifestyle, and try to live in an atmosphere of good humor. Be cheerful and forget your worries — and live longer.

Task One　Translation

Translate the underlined parts in the above sample into Chinese.

1) _____

_____

2) _____

_____

3) _____

_____

4) _____

_____

5) _____

Task Two　Writing

Suppose you have a friend who is ill and obsessed with some negative emotion. Write him a 200-word letter and give him some suggestions in line with the TCM theory on treating his disease and getting rid of the negative emotion. Try to use as many sentence patterns as possible in PART Ⅲ. Alternatively, you may work in pairs to do a role-play activity. One student acts as a doctor, giving TCM suggestions to the other student acting as a patient. Then exchange your roles. Search more information on the internet.

PART IV　REFLECTION

The preventative treatment theory is originally proposed in *Huangdi's Inner Canon of Medicine* and has been emphasized in China throughout the development of TCM. Actually, TCM has made great achievements in treating diseases before their onset and preventing diseases from exacerbating. Since 1996, WHO has made several yearly reports entitled "World Health Reports" (http://www.who.int/whr/previous/en/) advocating the importance of prevention.

Search the internet for information on **prevention and treatment of diseases** and think about the following questions:

1) Why does the entire medical field stress preventive work?

2) What are the benefits that TCM can offer in preventing and treating diseases?

Unit 6

Health Preservation in Traditional Chinese Medicine

LEARNING OUTCOMES

This unit offers you opportunities to:

- **explain** why and how medical qigong and Chinese medicinal cuisine promote health
- **introduce** the ways to preserve health in traditional Chinese medicine (TCM)
- **compare** different ways to preserve health in TCM
- **use** the terms related to health preservation in TCM
- **reflect on** the mass enthusiasm for health preservation nowadays

笔记

PART I　LISTENING AND SPEAKING

Before you listen

In this section you will hear a short passage entitled "Yoga and Traditional Chinese Medicine". The following words may be of help.

musculo-skeletal /ˌmʌskjʊləʊ ˈskelətl/	*a.*	肌肉骨骼的
intimately /ˈɪntɪmətli/	*ad.*	熟悉地；亲密地
energize /ˈenədʒaɪz/	*vt.*	给……以活力，使活跃
sluggish /ˈslʌgɪʃ/	*a.*	不活泼的；无精打采的
oriental /ˌɔːrɪˈent(ə)l/	*a.*	东方的；东方人的
soothing /ˈsuːðɪŋ/	*a.*	慰藉的；使人宽心的
pancreas /ˈpæŋkrɪəs/	*n.*	胰，胰腺
pharmacopeia /ˌfɑːməkəˈpiːə/	*n.*	处方汇编，药典
categorization /ˌkætəgəraɪˈzeɪʃ(ə)n/	*n.*	编目方法，分门别类

While you listen

Listen to the passage carefully and fill in each of the blanks marked from 1) to 10) according to what you have heard.

ER-6-1
Listening
practice

Yoga and Traditional Chinese Medicine

　　As we all know, acupuncture and moxibustion are used to treat specific diseases by unblocking stagnation in the organs and meridians, while yoga can be practiced to prevent diseases by keeping the meridians open and the qi or energy flowing.

　　The basic step in 1) ＿＿＿＿＿＿ health and healing disease is to release musculo-skeletal holding patterns which help deal with the internal physical and their 2) ＿＿＿＿＿＿ mental symptoms. This is the key to healing.

　　Specific yoga postures can 3) ＿＿＿＿＿＿ certain meridians. For instance, backbends 4) ＿＿＿＿＿＿ heat and energy to energize the yang aspect of the body, while forward bends emphasize the yin or cooling, and 5) ＿＿＿＿＿＿. If you feel cold or your reaction becomes much slower than normal, backbends will help you feel energetic by 6) ＿＿＿＿＿＿. The kidney is regarded as the "root" of yin and yang in traditional Chinese medicine. Similarly, Western medicine believes that the kidneys are the first 7) ＿＿＿＿＿＿ formed in the fetus.

　　If you are suffering insomnia or feeling energetic, 8) ＿＿＿＿＿＿ are a suitable choice for their soothing and calming effect 9) ＿＿＿＿＿＿ the yin aspect of the body. Right side bends and all twisting movements make stronger the liver and gallbladder,

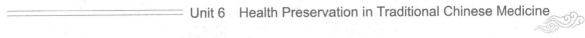

while left side bends make stronger the spleen and pancreas.

Yoga and acupuncture are 10) _____ in nature for their common aim of releasing stagnation of energy in the meridian system and their related organs or in the blood. While yoga may help relieve the blockage, acupuncture and meridian theory contribute to the understanding of the best poses for a particular condition. What's more, herbs can tonify and unblock stagnation.

After you listen

Please discuss with your partner the following questions and give your presentation to the class.

1) What is the difference between acupuncture and yoga in treating certain diseases?

2) Why do people practice yoga?

PART II　READING

Text A

An Introduction to Medical Qigong

1　Qigong is a system of Chinese health care that combines physical training, preventive and therapeutic medicine, with Eastern philosophy. The word "qi" (or *chi*) means air, breath of life, or vital essence. "*Gong*" means work, self-discipline, achievement or mastery. Qigong is said to be the cultivation and **deliberate** control of a higher form of vital energy, as well as an ancient philosophical system of harmonious **integration** of the human body with the universe. Qigong challenges the foundations of Western biomedical thought by rejecting the idea that the human species is unaffected by nature. More specifically, this art combines the physical benefits of **isometrics**, **isotonics**, and **aerobic** conditioning, with the healing elements of **meditation** and relaxation. Qigong is a **discipline** that focuses on gaining awareness and control over the life force or "qi" present in our bodies. There are more than 3,000 varieties of qigong, which can be divided into five major categories: Medical,[①] Daoist,[②] Buddhist,[③] Confucian,[④] and the Martial Arts.[⑤] Qigong is one of the soft forms[⑥] of a sub-set of disciplines that includes *taiji*, and the hard form[⑦] of kung fu. In this article, we will discuss medical qigong.

2　For many centuries, qigong has been a **mainstay** in Chinese medical practices. Ancient turtle-shell **artifacts** conclusively show the art was important at least 7,000 years ago. Archaeological evidence suggests the practice may date back one million years. About 2,000 years ago *Huangdi's Inner Canon of Medicine* was the first literature to systematically describe the tradition. In 1988, the Chinese held the first World Conference for exchanging qigong medical research in Beijing. Subsequent World Conferences took place in Tokyo and Berkeley. Another was held in the summer of 1996 in New York City.

3　North American psychological, physiological and medical researchers are also studying qigong with great interest. University students throughout North America have formed qigong groups. Even the film industry, with the creation of kung fu movies, has significantly increased the study's **proliferation**. Qigong homepages are blossoming on the Internet World Wide Web as well.

---

① Medical: 医家的,医家气功以防病治病、保健强身为主。
② Daoist: 道家的,道家气功重在修炼,以性命双修、修心炼性、清静无为为主。
③ Buddhist: 佛家的,佛家气功以悟性、炼心、超脱、空无和明心见性为主。
④ Confucian: 儒家的,儒家气功以摄生养气、存心养性为主。
⑤ Martial Arts: 武术,武家气功以御敌防身、提高技艺和表演为主。
⑥ soft forms:(气功的)软功,指用来养生健身的功夫,如太极拳、吐纳功、养生功等。
⑦ hard form:(气功的)硬功,指内强外壮、练气化力、抗暴制敌及强健筋骨的功夫。

4　Today, more than 70 million Chinese practice qigong daily. Some view the method as a curative step for existing **afflictions**, while others use the method as a preventative measure. Qigong can be an integral component in the fight against virtually any disease. As many as 50% of all diseases dismissed by **orthodox** doctors as untreatable or "**psychosomatic**" may be impressively impacted by the method; some of which are **eradicated** completely.

5　Chinese doctors have applied qigong in hospitals and clinics to treat individuals suffering from a variety of **maladies** such as constipation, insomnia and **gastritis**.

6　Since it is best used for **staving** off disease and treating chronic conditions or disabilities, qigong may not be the most suitable treatment for acute illness or medical emergencies. It can be used as a supplement to conventional medical practices. If one decides to try qigong during the course of treatment of an existing illness, it is advisable that one should do so under the guidance of a licensed Chinese medical doctor. Professional **supervision** is strongly suggested for beginners.

Preventing disease

7　In addition to its curative potential, by preventing the **onset** of disease, qigong can significantly reduce the amount of suffering and financial burden experienced by many patients due to long-term health care. Qigong increases physical strength, **heightens** resistance to infectious diseases and **premature senility,**[①] and helps ensure a long life. Practicing this method can greatly reduce the likelihood of **stroke**. It can improve blood sugar levels for diabetics. Because it normalizes the level of sex hormones, it helps ward off sexual **impotence** and **frigidity**. Practicing this discipline can hasten recovery from surgery as well as from sports and other injuries by up to 50%. Qigong offers individuals a way to achieve a relaxed, harmonious state of dynamic **equilibrium**. It typically improves overall health, allowing them to maintain a pain-free life full of vigor and grace.

How does qigong work?

8　Breathing and meditation[②] are an important part of medical qigong. In a qigong meditative state, one is fully relaxed, yet not in a **trance**. One can increase qi and direct it to any area of distress. Anxiety and self-doubt are replaced with peace of mind and increased confidence. Gradually, all distractions, worries, and hints of depression begin to dissipate. Meditation **fosters** feelings of happiness, which, in turn, stimulate circulation of blood and qi. This therapy contributes to the healing of those who are already ill as well as increasing the vitality of healthy individuals. People of all ages can develop and maintain internal vigor and good health through qigong.

9　Practicing qigong lowers blood pressure, pulse rates, metabolic rates, **lactate** production, and oxygen demand. It raises the endocrine system's capabilities. It also has

①　premature senility: 早衰,指与正常人相比提前衰老。

②　breathing and meditation: 呼吸(调息)与入静(调心)。呼吸是气功疗法的重要环节,通过锻炼,改胸式呼吸为腹式呼吸,改浅呼吸为深呼吸,最后练成自发的丹田呼吸。入静是指一种稳定的安静状态,无杂念,集中意念于一点,即意守丹田或留意呼吸,对外界刺激的感觉减弱。

a regulating effect on the substances: cyclic **adenosine monophosphate**① and cyclic **guanosine** monophosphate,② which play important roles in proper respiratory function and the delivery of oxygen to the body's cells. The sense of **serenity** the exercise produces is the result of slightly elevated body temperature and an increased rate of oxygen absorption. Qigong activates qi, improves blood circulation and balances yin and yang. It **bolster**s the immune system, and stimulates the conductivity of the meridians and channels through which qi flows.

10　The goal of qigong is to encourage the circulation of qi throughout the body. This helps the body resist or overcome imbalances or **blockages**. It shares similar objectives with some other disciplines such as acupuncture and Chinese herbal medicine. A primary aim of qigong is to maintain or restore balance and harmony of mind and body, while becoming aware of the human body's place within nature's oneness. As a qigong practitioner becomes more conscious of the state of his or her body, he or she gains a greater resistance to the imbalances and blockages affecting qi. This **sensitivity** aids in the balance of yin and yang, the two opposing forces of universal order. In the seventeenth century, Descartes③ **postulate** (which most Westerners still accept today) stated that mind and body are separate entities. The qigong student will contend that such a notion is a **fallacy**. It is in this context that we are able to understand the philosophy of qigong, where qi is the force that integrates the relationship between body (matter, structure) and mind (process, function). Scholars of this art gain more than improved health. They learn another way of viewing and experiencing the dynamic unity of life, an attitude far removed from the feelings of **disenchantment** and **alienation** common in Western civilization. Students of qigong learn to achieve their potential as highly successful members of our species.

How does one practice qigong?

11　One need not become a qigong master to experience many of its healing effects. For health purposes, one needs to learn only a few exercises. One must achieve a state of **tranquility**, find release from tension, take on a positive attitude and develop strong will power. Benefits can be further achieved in one of three ways. First, one can go to a master for treatment by that master's external qi.④ Although some masters exist in some Western **metropolitan** areas such as Chicago, New York, Los Angeles, San Francisco, or Vancouver, the most experienced masters reside in China. Second, one can seek education from a master and practice exercise and meditation. Third, in a supervised group, one can

---

① cyclic adenosine monophosphate: 环磷酸腺苷,是细胞内参与调节物质代谢和生物学功能的重要物质,是生命信息传递的"第二信使"。

② cyclic guanosine monophosphate: 环磷酸鸟苷,是一种具有细胞内信息传递作用的第二信使,可被 G 蛋白偶联受体(G-protein linked receptor)激活的蛋白激酶(protein kinases)活化,进而将细胞外信号传导至细胞核。

③ Descartes: 勒内·笛卡尔,法国哲学家、数学家、物理学家。他对现代数学的发展做出了重要的贡献,被称为"解析几何之父"。他还是西方现代哲学思想的奠基人,是近代唯物论的开拓者。他提出了"普遍怀疑"的主张,又被称为"现代哲学之父"。

④ external qi: 外气,即气功师发布于体外的"气",是以能量(物质)为载体的生命信息,是一种生物能场。

learn to treat oneself. The latter is the most realistic option for most people.

12 In order to fully benefit from qigong training, one must apply time, patience, determination and persistence. This art involves more than simple physical training. It requires retraining one's breathing and thought processes. Learning the basics can take from three months to a year. As with any other human **endeavor**, some people will prove more **adept** at the art than others, and so will progress more quickly. However, anyone with enough motivation can learn adequate skills to make a positive impact upon one's quality of life. While there are no shortcuts, there are also no limits to how far one may progress.

Reference: GUO Y Q. An introduction to medical qigong [EB/OL]. [2015-10-05]. http://acupuncture. com/newsletters/m_aug06/main1.htm.

New words

deliberate /dɪˈlɪb(ə)rət/	*a.*	done consciously and intentionally 故意的；蓄意的
integration /ˌɪntɪˈɡreɪʃ(ə)n/	*n.*	the act or process of combining two or more things so that they work together 结合，整合
isometrics /ˌaɪsə(ʊ)ˈmetrɪks/	*n.*	(*pl.*) a system of physical exercises in which muscles are caused to act against each other or against a fixed object 静力锻炼法
isotonics /ˌaɪsə(ʊ)ˈtɒnɪks/	*n.*	muscular exercise using free weights or fixed devices to simulate resistance of weight 等张（力）训练
aerobic /eəˈrəʊbɪk/	*a.*	relating to, involving, or requiring free oxygen 需氧的，有氧的
meditation /ˌmedɪˈteɪʃ(ə)n/	*n.*	the practice of thinking deeply in silence, especially for religious reasons or in order to make your mind calm 沉思，冥想
discipline /ˈdɪsɪplɪn/	*n.*	a branch of knowledge, typically one studied in higher education 学科
mainstay /ˈmeɪnsteɪ/	*n.*	sth. on which sth. else is based or relies 主要支柱
artifact /ˈɑːtɪfækt/	*n.*	an object made by a human being, typically one of cultural or historical interest 人工制品，手工艺品
proliferation /ˌprəlɪfəˈreɪʃn/	*n.*	rapid increase in the number or amount of sth. 激增；剧增

笔记

affliction /əˈflɪkʃ(ə)n/	n.	a cause of pain or harm 苦恼，痛苦
orthodox /ˈɔːθədɒks/	a.	following or conforming to the traditional or generally accepted rules or beliefs of a religion, philosophy, or practice 规范的；正统的
psychosomatic /ˌsaɪkə(ʊ)səˈmætɪk/	a.	(of a physical illness or other condition) caused or aggravated by a mental factor such as internal conflict or stress 受心理影响的
eradicate /ɪˈrædɪkeɪt/	vt.	destroy completely; put an end to 摧毁；完全根除
malady /ˈmælədi/	n.	a disease or ailment 疾病，病症
gastritis /gæˈstraɪtɪs/	n.	inflammation of the lining of the stomach 胃炎
stave /steɪv/	vi.	avert or delay sth. bad or dangerous 避免，延缓
supervision /ˌsuːpəˈvɪʒn/	n.	the work or activity involved in being in charge of sb./sth. and making sure that everything is done correctly, safely, etc. 监督；管理
onset /ˈɒnset/	n.	the beginning of sth., especially sth. unpleasant 开始
heighten /ˈhaɪt(ə)n/	vt.	make or become more intense（使）变高，（使）加强
premature /ˈpremətʃə/	a.	occurring or done before the usual or proper time; too early 过早的，提前的
senility /sɪˈnɪlɪti/	n.	behaving in a confused or strange way, and being unable to remember things, because you are old 衰老的状态
stroke /strəʊk/	n.	a sudden disabling attack or loss of consciousness caused by an interruption in the flow of blood to the brain, especially through thrombosis 脑卒中
impotence /ˈɪmpət(ə)ns/	n.	inability in a man to achieve an erection or orgasm 阳痿
frigidity /frɪˈdʒɪdɪti/	n.	(in a woman) the lack of the ability to enjoy sex（尤指妇女的）性感缺失，性冷淡
equilibrium /ˌiːkwɪˈlɪbrɪəm/	n.	a state in which opposing forces or influences are balanced 平衡

笔记

trance /trɑːns/	n.	a half-conscious state characterized by an absence of response to external stimuli, typically as induced by hypnosis(催眠) or entered by a medium 出神；恍惚
foster /ˈfɒstə/	vt.	encourage the development of (sth., especially sth. desirable) 培养；促进
lactate /ˈlækteɪt/	n.	a salt or ester of lactic acid 乳酸
adenosine /əˈdenə(ʊ)siːn/	n.	a compound consisting of adenine(腺嘌呤) combined with ribose(核糖), present in all living tissue in combined form as nucleotides 腺苷
monophosphate /ˌmɒnəˈfɒsfeɪt/	n.	a chemical composition that only has one phosphate group 一磷酸盐
guanosine /ˈgwɑːnəsiːn/	n.	a compound consisting of guanine combined with ribose, present in all living tissue in combined form as nucleotides 鸟苷，鸟嘌呤核苷
serenity /sɪˈrenɪti/	n.	the state of being calm, peaceful, and untroubled 宁静，平静
bolster /ˈbəʊlstə/	vt.	support or strengthen 支持，支撑
blockage /ˈblɒkɪdʒ/	n	an obstruction which makes movement or flow difficult or impossible 堵塞，阻滞
sensitivity /ˌsensɪˈtɪvɪti/	n.	the ability to understand other people's feelings 敏感；灵敏性
postulate /ˈpɒstjʊleɪt/	n.	a thing suggested or assumed as true as the basis for reasoning, discussion, or belief 假定，基本原理
fallacy /ˈfæləsi/	n.	a mistaken belief, especially one based on unsound arguments 谬误，谬论
disenchantment /ˌdɪs(ɪ)nˈtʃɑːntm(ə)nt/	n.	a feeling of disappointment about sb. or sth. you previously respected or admired; disillusionment 觉醒，清醒
alienation /ˌeɪlɪəˈneɪʃ(ə)n/	n.	the act of making somebody less friendly or sympathetic towards you 离间，疏远
tranquility /træŋˈkwɪlɪti/	n.	the state of being quiet and peaceful 平静，安静
metropolitan /ˌmetrəˈpɒlɪt(ə)n/	a.	connected with a large or capital city 大都会的，大城市的
endeavor /ɪnˈdevə/	n.	an attempt to achieve a goal　努力，尽力

adept /əˈdept/　　　　　　　　*a.*　　very skilled or proficient at something 精于……的,擅长于……的

Phrases and expressions

vital essence	精华
vital energy	生命力,气
aerobic conditioning	有氧运动
turtle-shell artifact	龟甲制品
preventative measure	预防措施
stave off	延缓;推迟
chronic condition	慢性病
acute illness	急性病
medical emergency	急诊
curative potential	治愈潜能
physical strength	体力
infectious disease	传染病
blood sugar level	血糖水平
ward off	预防
dynamic equilibrium	动态平衡
internal vigor	机体活力
metabolic rate	代谢率
imbalance and blockage	失衡和阻滞
balance of yin and yang	阴阳平衡,阴平阳秘
reside in	居住,存在于
be adept at	擅长,善于

Task One　Preview

1. Learn the following roots and affixes. Write out the Chinese meaning of the given words.

Roots/ Affixes	Meaning of roots/affixes	Words	Chinese meaning of the given words
art-/arti-	skill	artifact	_____
		artificial	_____
equ	equal, same	equal	_____
		equilibrium	_____
fibr (o)	fiber	fibroblast	_____
		fibroma	_____

immun (o)	immunity	immunology	_____
		immunotherapy	_____
iso-	equal	isometric	_____
		isotonic	_____
ject	throw	project	_____
		reject	_____
mega-	large	megacardia	_____
		megalocyte	_____
metro-	mother	metropolis	_____
		metropolitan	_____
orth (o)-	straight, upright	orthodox	_____
		orthoepy	_____
poly-	many	polyplegia	_____
		polyuria	_____
potent	power, ability	impotence	_____
		potential	_____
psych (o)	mind	psychosis	_____
		psychotherapy	_____
sphygm (o)	pulse	sphygmometer	_____
		sphygmogram	_____
steth (o)	chest	stethography	_____
		stethoscope	_____
vascul (o)	blood vessel	vascular	_____
		vasculature	_____
ven (o)	vein	venogram	_____
		venous	_____

2. Write down the questions you would like to ask or discuss about the text.

_____

_____

_____

Task Two　Speaking

1. Answer the following questions according to the text.

1) How do the practitioners benefit from qigong?

2) What categories can qigong be divided into?

3) In what cases is qigong not suggested as a therapy?

4) What role does qigong play in preventing diseases?

5) What contributions does meditation make to the people practicing qigong?

6) Why do the practitioners of qigong have the sense of serenity?

7) What is the primary aim of practicing qigong?

8) For common people, in what ways can they achieve benefits from practicing qigong and what is the most realistic way for them?

2. Work in pairs or groups and exchange views on the following passage.

Traditional Chinese Medicine at Home

Traditional Chinese medicine (TCM) has been widely used in China for thousands of years. Today it has spread around the world to help people cure illnesses and prevent health problems. Besides treatment for physical and mental ailments by physicians, you can use TCM by yourself at home to ensure a healthier and happier life.

First, keep balanced diet. Balanced diet is optimal for health. The food that you eat will become your body's energy because it contains important nutrients, vitamins and minerals. Include as many fruits and vegetables as possible into your diet. Cut down on the amount of sugar and salt as well as fatty and spicy food in your diet, and try to avoid refined flours and products as well as caffeine and alcohol.

Second, do exercises. TCM states that activity is vital to proper health. Do some exercises in your daily routines. You can do them at home, workplace, or the gym. You can walk to workplace rather than driving. Exercises are beneficial to both physical and mental wellbeing.

Third, drink tea. Tea has always been a curative and beneficial drink in China. The natural chemicals in tea have been found to be really good for health. Tea also has antioxidant(抗氧化剂)properties. Many herbal teas are easily available on the market and can be drunk anytime at home.

Fourth, take herbal therapy. Many TCM herbs can be taken at home. Some can be used when you are feeling a bit under the weather, while others can be used regularly to prevent diseases. You can buy capsules containing several pre-mixed herbs for convenience.

The above are just a few things that you can do at home, at work, or any place at any time. By incorporating TCM into your daily life, you can have a greater sense of wellbeing.

Topic for discussion: What do you learn from the passage in terms of incorporating TCM into your daily life?

Task Three　Vocabulary

1. Match up each word in Column A with its appropriate definition from Column B.

Column A	Column B
1) affliction	a. a sudden serious illness when a blood vessel in the brain bursts or is blocked
2) gastritis	b. a serious problem
3) tranquility	c. (of a disease) lasting for a long time; difficult to cure or get rid of

4) infectious

   d. a serious, unexpected, and often dangerous situation requiring immediate action

5) meditation

   e. a mistaken belief, especially one based on unsound arguments

6) emergency

   f. behaving in a confused or strange way, and being unable to remember things, because you are old

7) metabolism

   g. an illness in which the inside of the stomach becomes swollen and painful

8) chronic

9) senility

   h. pain and suffering or sth. that causes it

   i. liable to be transmitted to people, organisms, etc. through the environment

10) fallacy

   j. the chemical processes in living things that change food, etc. into energy and materials for growth

11) stroke

   k. the state of being quiet and peaceful

12) malady

   l. the practice of thinking deeply in silence, especially for religious reasons or in order to make your mind calm

2. Fill in the blanks with the words given below. Change the form where necessary.

form	advance	invade	mild	somehow
appearance	somewhat	cultivate	link	exterior
emotion	therefore	chronic	nurture	otherwise

Preventive Principles in Traditional Chinese Medicine

Traditional Chinese medicine (TCM) has been always attaching great importance to prevention. The earliest preventive thought, known as "curing a disease before its onset" was 1) _____ in *Huangdi's Inner Cannon of Medicine*. It has imposed great influence on the 2) _____ and development of preventive medicine.

Various measures should be taken in advance to prevent the onset of diseases, including health preservation and prevention of the 3) _____ by pathogenic factors. Health preservation includes complying with nature, 4) _____ mental faculties, balancing work and rest, having proper diet and living habits. To prevent the invasion of pathogenic factors, the following three aspects should be followed: first, pay attention to hygiene to prevent environmental, water and food pollution; second, avoid the invasion by pathogenic factors such as six excesses, seven 5) _____ , and improper diet; third, try to avoid all kinds of injuries.

Early treatment of a disease is easy because it is 6) _____ and the healthy qi has not declined yet. If not treated timely, disease will become complicated and worse because of the transmission of pathogenic qi from the 7) _____ into the interior and the exhaustion of healthy qi. Therefore, early diagnosis and treatment are essential to recovery and the prevention of disease transmission, development and aggravation.

笔记

Cutting off the transmission 8) _____ of a disease is a major way to prevent the development and aggravation of the condition.

When disease is 9) _____ relieved, probably it may recur due to improper diet, emotional disturbance, etc. For instance, when just recovering from diarrhea, infants should have light food; 10) _____, heavy diet and overeating will impair the functions of the spleen and stomach and result in the recurrence of disease.

Task Four　Translation

1. Study the following sentences and pay attention to the underlined parts.

1) Qigong is a system of Chinese health care that <u>combines</u> physical training, preventive and therapeutic medicine, <u>with</u> Eastern philosophy. (para. 1)

2) Qigong is a discipline that <u>focuses on</u> gaining awareness and control over the life force or "qi" present in our bodies. (para.1)

3) Archaeological evidence suggests the practice may <u>date back</u> one million years. (para. 2)

4) If one decides to try qigong during the course of treatment of an existing illness, <u>it is advisable that</u> one should do so under the guidance of a licensed Chinese medical doctor. (para. 6)

5) This therapy <u>contributes to</u> the healing of those who are already ill as well as increasing the vitality of healthy individuals. (para. 8)

6) It also <u>has</u> a regulating <u>effect on</u> the substances: cyclic adenosine monophosphate and cyclic guanosine monophosphate, which <u>play important roles in</u> proper respiratory function and the delivery of oxygen to the body's cells. (para. 9)

7) <u>It is</u> in this context <u>that</u> we are able to understand the philosophy of qigong, where qi is the force that integrates the relationship between body (matter, structure) and mind (process, function). (para. 10)

8) However, anyone with enough motivation can learn adequate skills to <u>make a positive impact upon</u> one's quality of life. (para. 12)

2. Translate the following sentences into English.

1) 一名优秀的医生应该将高超的医术与高尚的医德有机结合起来。

2) 练习气功时,应该将注意力集中在呼吸上,将气引导至身体的任何不适之处。

3) 用醋抗感染和其他急性疾病的做法可追溯至希波克拉底时代(公元前 460–377)。

4) 你患上了急性肺炎,建议你住院接受治疗。

5) 据说,医疗事故导致她病情恶化,最终死亡。

6) 随着科学技术的发展,医疗设备在预防和治疗疾病过程中发挥着越来越重要的作用。

7) 正是通过坚持体育锻炼,他逐渐增强了体力,提高了身体对传染性疾病的抵抗力,实现了延年益寿的愿望。

8) 长期大量服用药物会对健康造成不良影响。

Text B

Chinese Medicinal Cuisine[①]

1　A lot of people all over the world like to eat Chinese food, but Chinese medicinal **cuisine** (Chinese food therapy) is an ancient healing art. It is a kind of traditional medicine.

2　Long ago, people taught about how the body operated and gave suggestions about what to prepare to stay healthy or cure disease. If you are interested in exploring traditional Chinese cooking methods for better health, here is some background information, general principles, and **recipes**.

3　The common Chinese food eaten around the world isn't **authentic** though. Authentic Chinese food dishes are prepared according to traditional recipes and techniques, based on ancient ideas about how the human body operates, and they described the effect of each kind of meat, grain, herb, or vegetable on the human body.

History of medicinal cuisine

4　Ancient Chinese medical books list hundreds of plants, animals and chemical **ingredients** and tell their specific effects on the human body. These books give ideas about the physical principles involved in human health, and they describe how herbs or special foods help people, along with medical techniques such as moxibustion and acupuncture.

5　The earliest work on these topics dates from the early Han Dynasty (206 BC-220 AD) and is called *Huangdi's Inner Canon of Medicine*. It is more than 2,000 years old. Though that was very long ago, it contains the basic ideas of Chinese food therapy. It classifies food into four groups and five tastes by their natures and characteristics. The text gives recommendations on what to eat for different health conditions and different environmental conditions. It explains what to eat in different environments such as cold weather, hot weather, rainy or dry conditions, and what to eat in specific medical conditions.

6　Since that time, the basic ideas about food and health have changed little.

General principles of Chinese medicinal cooking

7　Keep balance. The basic idea is to balance the qi, yin and yang and the body fluids. This is also the basic TCM idea. It is thought that a healthy body or organ has a proper balance of these things. When they are out of balance, there is disease or sickness.

8　The environmental or physical injury disrupts the balance. For example, cold weather causes a lack of yang qi or high yin in the body. So high yang foods are eaten. In hot weather when there is naturally too much yang, high yin foods are eaten.

---

① Chinese medicinal cuisine: 指中国药膳。

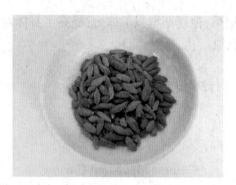

9　Add medicinal herbs to your diet. Healing herbs or animal parts can be added to the diet to build up health. Many of the same herbs are used by Western herbalists and herbalists in other parts of the world for the same conditions, so this strongly suggests that the herbs have real medicinal effects. Otherwise, how did people all over the world have the same herbal treatment ideas for hundreds of years?

10　Mix heats and flavors. All foods are **categorized** by the nature or property, ranging from high yang to high yin, and one of the five food flavors (sour, sweet, bitter, pungent and salty).[①] A food item's property and specific flavor influences the body in its own way.

11　It is thought that people should generally include all the flavors in every meal and balance the temperatures. So generally a healthy meal will include both yin and yang food items and each of these five tastes. In main **stir-fried** dishes, a variety of ingredients with each of these **attributes** are usually mixed and fried together.

12　Most Chinese people think that if too much of one type of food is consumed, an imbalance may arise in the body.

Seasonal recipes

13　It is interesting that the Chinese believe that eating seasonal food is generally the best. For example, in the summer, yin foods like **melons** and cucumber are available; and in the winter, high yang foods like **garlic** and onions are available for consumption as well as easily stored red pepper and other high yang herbs. The following recipes use common ingredients that you can make for each season for the year.

　　Winter: Chicken and **Ginger** Soup Recipe

14　Just like Westerners, Chinese people like to drink lots of hot soup on cold winter days. The purpose is to make soups with high yang vegetables and herbs, including meat to balance the dish. A favorite winter soup, just like in the West, is chicken soup.

15　Take chicken portions and boil them together with two **chopped** potatoes, or half a *bailuobo* (the long white Chinese turnip), and one tablespoon of ginger. When the potato and chicken pieces are somewhat cooked, add **diced** vegetables and spices.

16　The diced vegetables should include three diced cloves of garlic and one chopped onion, since these are essential for adding yang. You can also include a cup of carrots, a

---

①　the five food flavors (sour, sweet, bitter, pungent and salty): 食物的五味，具体包括酸、甘、苦、辛、咸。

cup of mushrooms, or other similar vegetables.

17   To the mix, add one teaspoon of sea salt and add additional herbs such as several thin-sliced pieces of *Huangqi*, or pinches of **turmeric**, if you wish. If you like red pepper, add it!

Spring: **Asparagus** and Vinegar Recipe

18   In the spring, things come alive and start growing. It is important for living things to have more than usual yang for growth.

19   As the saying goes, "green is the color of the liver and of spring."[1] It is advised to eat fresh leafy greens and sprouts that are available, and drink fresh sour juices, since these stimulate qi.

20   It is also thought to be a time when the body does a "spring cleaning" on itself by getting rid of stored fats and meat, so eating less meat and fat is considered to be better for health. Here is a light and easy-to-make **vegetarian** dish and drink that is a good example of a springtime meal.

21   Wash a bunch of asparagus and a carrot in clean water without **detergent**. Then chop up the vegetables and lightly steam them until the asparagus is slightly tender and bright green. Note that the vegetables cook quickly so don't steam them long.

22   Prepare a dressing by simply adding about two parts of virgin olive oil to one part of plum vinegar or apple cider vinegar. Plum vinegar is preferred because it is a springtime fruit. Then pour the dressing on the vegetables and enjoy the dish with some **lemonade**. To make the lemonade, simply **squeeze** a fresh lemon and add the juice to clean water.

Summer: Tomato and Cucumber Salad Recipe

23   Here is a favorite dish for summer when the yang is naturally high, and you need to cool down a bit. Tomato and cucumber are high yin vegetables that are readily available.

24   Try to find fresh and ripe ingredients. Dice some red onion, or if that is unavailable, dice a regular onion and chop up tomatoes and cucumbers. Mix up the ingredients with virgin olive oil, and add some dill, salt, and pepper to taste. It is simple to make and great for hot summer days.

Autumn: Butternut Squash Soup Recipe

25   In the autumn, life naturally ebbs away, and it is thought that the qi returns to the earth. In the human body, the qi goes inwards into the body's core.[2]

26   Eating the vegetables and fruits that are available at these times helps your body to transition and stay healthy. Here is a recipe for butternut squash soup, but pumpkin or other kinds of squash can be substituted.

27   Take a large butternut squash or an equivalently-sized pumpkin or other squash, a medium onion, two cloves of garlic, a stalk of **celery**, a large carrot, some boiled chicken

---

①   Green is the color of the liver and of spring: 青为肝与春之主色。中医学认为,五色(即青、赤、黄、白、黑)与五脏(肝、心、脾、肺、肾)相应,也与五季(春、夏、长夏、秋、冬)相应。故五色为其相应脏腑或季节的主色。

②   the qi goes inwards into the body's core: 秋季气开始在体内蛰伏。

meat, and salt, pepper, **cinnamon**, and **nutmeg** to taste.

28　Chop up and dice everything, and first boil the squash in water in a large pot. Then when the squash is almost done, add the rest of the vegetables and the already cooked chicken chunks, and simmer the soup for a few minutes. Then when the soup is ready, cool it a little while, add in the spice and mix it well.

　　Reference: Chinese medicinal cuisine [EB/OL]. [2015-10-05]. http://www.chinahighlights.com/travelguide/chinese-food/medicinal-cuisine.htm.

New words

cuisine /kwɪˈziːn/	*n.*	a style or method of cooking, especially as characteristic of a particular country, region, or establishment 烹饪；菜肴
recipe /ˈresɪpi/	*n.*	a set of instructions for preparing a particular dish, including a list of the ingredients required 食谱
authentic /ɔːˈθentɪk/	*a.*	of undisputed origin and not a copy; genuine 真正的，真实的
ingredient /ɪnˈgriːdɪənt/	*n.*	any of the foods or substances that are combined to make a particular dish（烹调的）原料
categorize /ˈkætəgəraɪz/	*vt.*	place in a particular class or group 把……归类，把……分门别类
stir-fry /ˈstə: fraɪ/	*vt.*	fry (meat, fish, or vegetables) rapidly over a high heat while stirring briskly 用旺火煸，用旺火炒
attribute /ˈætrɪbjuːt/	*n.*	a quality or feature regarded as a characteristic or inherent part of sb. or sth. 品质，特征
melon /ˈmelən/	*n.*	the large round fruit of a plant of the gourd family, with sweet pulpy flesh and many seeds 甜瓜
garlic /ˈgɑːlɪk/	*n.*	a strong-smelling pungent-tasting bulb, used as flavoring in cooking and in herbal medicine 大蒜；蒜头
ginger /ˈdʒɪndʒə/	*n.*	a hot, fragrant spice made from the rhizome（根茎）of a plant, which may be chopped or powdered for cooking, preserved in syrup, or candied 生姜

chop /tʃɔp/	vt.	cut (sth.) into pieces with repeated sharp blows of an axe or knife 切碎，砍
dice /daɪs/	vt.	cut (food or other matter) into small cubes 将……切成丁
turmeric /ˈtəːmərɪk/	n.	a bright yellow aromatic powder obtained from the rhizome of a plant of the ginger family, used for flavoring and coloring in Asian cooking and formerly as a fabric dye 姜黄
asparagus /əˈspærəgəs/	n.	a tall plant of the lily family with fine feathery foliage（叶子）, cultivated for its edible shoots 芦笋
vegetarian /ˌvedʒɪˈteərɪən/	n.	a person who does not eat meat or fish, and sometimes other animal products, especially for moral, religious, or health reasons 素食者
detergent /dɪˈtəːdʒ(ə)nt/	n.	a water-soluble cleansing agent which combines with impurities and dirt to make them more soluble, and differs from soap in not forming a scum（浮沫）with the salts in hard water 洗涤剂；去垢剂
lemonade /ˌleməˈneɪd/	n.	a drink made from lemon juice and water sweetened with sugar 柠檬汽水，柠檬饮料
squeeze /skwiːz/	vt.	firmly press (sth. soft or yielding), typically with one's fingers 挤，榨
celery /ˈseləri/	n.	a cultivated plant of the parsley family, with closely packed succulent（多汁的）leaf stalks which are used as a salad or cooked vegetable 芹菜
cinnamon /ˈsɪnəmən/	n.	an aromatic spice made from the peeled, dried, and rolled bark of a SE Asian tree 肉桂
nutmeg /ˈnʌtmeg/	n.	the hard, aromatic, almost spherical seed of a tropical tree 肉豆蔻

Phrases and expressions

| medicinal cuisine | 药膳 |
| food therapy | 食疗 |

笔记

general principle	基本原则
out of balance	失衡,失调
medicinal effect	药用效果
in its own way	按其自身的方式
be essential for	对……来说重要
come alive	活跃起来
chop up	切细,切断
cool down	冷却;平静下来
ebb away	渐渐衰退;消逝

Task One　Preview

1. Learn the following roots and affixes. Write out the Chinese meaning of the given words.

Roots/ Affixes	Meaning of roots/affixes	Words	Chinese meaning of the given words
-ade	forming a noun	arcade	_____
		blockade	_____
brach (i)	arm	brachial	_____
		brachialis	_____
cauli	caudex	cauliflower	_____
		caulis	_____
cise	cut	incise	_____
		excise	_____
coron	crown	coronary	_____
		coronation	_____
cuis/cuit	cook	cuisine	_____
		biscuit	_____
-gen	that which produces	glycogen	_____
		pathogen	_____
gluco	relating to glucose	glucocorticoid	_____
		glucoprotein	_____
hemo/haemato	relating to blood	hematoma	_____
		hemoglobin	_____
hetero-	different	heterogeneous	_____
		heterosexual	_____
hypno	relating to sleep	hypnotherapy	_____
		hypnotics	_____

mal-	in a faulty or inadequate manner	malfunction	_____
		malnutrition	_____
nulli	none	nullify	_____
		nulliparous	_____
sinus (o)	sinus, cavity	sinuses	_____
		sinusitis	_____
-tension	pressure	hypertension	_____
		hypotension	_____
uni-	one	unilateral	_____
		uniline	_____
valv (o)	valve	valved	_____
		valvular	_____
vege	plant	vegetable	_____
		vegetarian	_____

2. Write down the questions you would like to ask or discuss about the text.

_____

_____

_____

Task Two　Vocabulary

Choose the word or phrase that can best complete the statements.

1) The eyes of some fish have a greater _____ to light than those of human beings do.

　A. sensitivity　　　B. longevity　　　C. serenity　　　D. irritability

2) In TCM, _____ may be practiced both as a still form with no physical movement and as a moving form, such as in qigong.

　A. transportation　　B. medication　　C. meditation　　D. respiration

3) Because of terrible injury, her playing career had to come to a _____ end in 2008.

　A. prevalent　　　B. premature　　　C. precise　　　D. previous

4) Eating this kind of fruit and some physical exercises often _____ the risks of heart disease.

　A. produce　　　B. reproduce　　　C. enhance　　　D. reduce

5) In China, Western medicine is often regarded as more effective in emergent situations, while TCM is more effective for immune conditions or _____ illness.

　A. chronic　　　B. acute　　　C. ironic　　　D. urgent

6) Vitamins and minerals are essential for the proper growth and _____ of a living organism.

　A. metabolism　　B. stagnation　　C. density　　　D. stasis

7) Phlegm _____ when the lungs are irritated, and when the moisture of the body is

overheated by pathogenic qi.

    A. stimulates   B. discharges   C. accumulates   D. secretes

8) He is suffering from digestive _____ caused by depression.

    A. impairment   B. sensation   C. alienation   D. dysfunction

9) When qi is deficient and unable to maintain sufficient and smooth blood circulation, the patient will have palpitations, chest tightness, _____ sweating and shortness of breath.

    A. rebellious   B. spontaneous   C. infectious   D. endogenous

10) A(n) _____ in certain chemicals leads to disturbances in the brain's function.

    A. imbalance   B. retention   C. depletion   D. circulation

11) TCM intervention could effectively control and _____ the symptoms and prevent the disease from exacerbation (恶化).

    A. transfer   B. descend   C. decrease   D. alleviate

12) Qigong can also _____ chronic pain, and help to treat depression and even some severe diseases such as cancer and diabetes.

    A. conceive   B. deceive   C. relieve   D. receive

13) Acupuncture is one of the most _____ forms of alternative therapy, which helps treat a variety of ailments.

    A. active   B. effective   C. sensitive   D. integrative

14) The principle of qigong rests in the idea of controlling and _____ qi to cure illnesses, produce a sense of well-being and even develop extraordinary abilities such as withstanding hard blows to the body.

    A. manipulating   B. adjusting   C. combining   D. promoting

15) Chinese food therapy is based on the well-known fact that improper eating leads to illnesses and proper diet _____ to the body's health.

    A. distributes   B. attributes   C. contributes   D. constitutes

Task Three   Translation

Translate the following expressions into English.

1) 养生康复   2) 导引

3) 吐纳   4) 恬淡虚无

5) 疏风解表   6) 法于阴阳，和于术数

7) 形与神俱   8) 精神内守

9) 积精全神   10) 延年益寿

11) 饮食偏嗜   12) 认知疗法

13) 因时制宜   14) 增强体力

15) 防止早衰   16) 保持动态平衡

17) 刺激气血循环   18) 维持机体活力和健康

19) 克服失调或阻滞   20) 恢复身心平衡和协调

PART III　TRANSLATION AND WRITING

How to Introduce the Exercises for Health Preservation

There are many traditional exercises for health preservation in TCM, for example, qigong, *taijiquan*, and *daoyin*. To introduce these exercises, one needs to include the following details: 1) the brief history of the exercise(简要历史); 2) people suitable to practice (适宜群体); 3) main features of the exercise (主要特点); 4) benefits of practicing (练习的好处); 5) suggestions of practicing the exercise (练习的建议); and 6) requirements of practicing the exercise(练习的要求).

The following sentences or expressions are commonly used to introduce *baduanjin* (Eight-section Brocade).

1) *Baduanjin* is a kind of body-building qigong with physical and mental care function which circulates widely in Chinese folk culture.

八段锦是一种中国民间流传广泛的、具有身心保健作用的健身气功。

2) *Baduanjin*, which represents the Chinese traditional physical exercise, is popular among the people because of its long history and excellent health care effect.

以八段锦为代表的中国传统体育运动，凭借其悠久的历史、卓越的医疗保健功效，为人民群众所喜爱，广为流传。

3) In China, everyone knows radio gymnastic exercises, but seldom knows it comes from *baduanjin*, which is a set of medical and healing exercises created by ancient people.

在中国，大家都知道广播体操，但是很少有人知道广播体操起源于八段锦，即古人创编的一套医疗、康复体操。

4) As far as old people are concerned, they may select some simple, easy and effective exercises like *baduanjin* to promote the functional activities of qi of the human body.

对于老年人来说，可以选择简单、易行、有效的保健运动，如八段锦，以促进气机在体内的生发。

5) Practicing *baduanjin* is helpful to strengthen the heart and lung functions, keep body appearance and increase the body qualities for young people.

练习八段锦有助于年轻人增强心肺功能，保持体形，提高身体素质。

6) For coronary heart disease (CHD) patients in the community, apart from conventional therapy, *baduanjin* can be popularized as an important supplementary rehabilitative means, which is simple, easy, effective and cheap.

对于社区冠心病患者，除了接受常规治疗，还可以推广具有简、便、验、廉特点的八段锦运动，作为重要的补充康复手段。

7) *Baduanjin* is safe, inexpensive, and easy to do, and can be integrated as part of a daily exercise regimen that can reduce stress from a hectic lifestyle.

八段锦安全、价廉、方便，可以与日常锻炼融为一体，从而减轻忙碌的生活方式所带来的压力。

8) *Baduanjin* can relieve the anxious and depressive mental state of CHD (coronary heart disease) patients.

八段锦运动能够改善冠心病患者焦虑和抑郁的心理状态。

9) *Baduanjin* is one kind of qigong that trains the neck, shoulder, back, chest, arm, and leg in order to warm up all parts of the body to gain health.

八段锦是气功的形式之一，可以锻炼颈部、肩部、背部、胸部、手臂和腿部，从而使全身各部活动开来，以获得健康。

10) People learn to control their limbs and body better, and the crouching stances help to develop stronger legs.

人们学习更好地控制四肢和身体，蹲伏姿势有助于将双腿锻炼得更为强壮。

11) In *baduanjin* exercise, the diaphragm moves up and down, doing internal massage of the organs and producing secretions which improve digestion and other metabolisms.

练习八段锦时，膈膜上下运动，对脏腑内部进行按摩，产生分泌物，从而促进消化和其他新陈代谢。

12) Each group practices *baduanjin* 50 minutes every morning following the instructors.

各组每日清晨在带教老师带领下练习八段锦50分钟。

13) If you are suffering from an ailment and already consult a physician, it is wise to inform your doctor about your interest in *baduanjin* and discuss how it can affect your treatment program.

如果你身患疾病，而且已经就医，那么告诉医生你对八段锦感兴趣，并且讨论练习八段锦会如何影响治疗方案也是一种明智的做法。

14) Do not practice *baduanjin* within one hour after a big meal or a half hour after a small meal.

在饱餐后一小时之内或者少餐后半小时之内，不要练习八段锦。

15) In order to have any beneficial effect on your health, it is very important to practice *baduanjin* with confidence, sincerity and perseverance.

为有益健康，练习八段锦务必满怀信心，真心诚意，坚持不懈。

Sample

Baduanjin

Baduanjin was developed during the twelfth century by the famous general Yueh Fei as a way to strengthen the body, to balance the vital functions and to drive stagnant energy and toxins from the system. 1) *Baduanjin* is a very popular qigong set, ideal for beginners. By involving your mind in your qigong practice you will get their full benefits. But, even by practicing the set as simple physical exercises, 2) the *Baduanjin* routine will loosen your muscles, improve your posture, enhance your blood circulation, and relax you.

There are various styles of the eight pieces. They are designed to help people to balance energy. 3) Most of the eight movements begin with drawing energy up with the movement of the hands and arms, and then pressing it back down. The movements have no beginning or end, but generally take the following cycle.

- Balanced and centered, aware of the whole body.
- Keep the body relaxed. So do the eyes, open and soft.
- Keep the elbows and knees and wrists relaxed even when you need to extend the limbs.
- Let energy flow through the body and move the body in a natural way.
- Inhale through the nose and exhale through the mouth. Breathe in a natural and gentle way. 4) Let your breath lead your movement. The body "rides" the breath.

Generally, one does the set once a day, with six, nine, or twelve repetitions of each movement. 5) If you do these movements once a day, you can build up gradually, starting with three repetitions for a couple of weeks, then six, then nine, and eventually twelve.

Task One   Translation

Translate the underlined parts in the above sample into Chinese.

1) _____

_____

2) _____

_____

3) _____

_____

4) _____

_____

5) _____

_____

Task Two   Writing

Choose a method of health preservation in traditional Chinese medicine and write a 200-word introduction to it. Try to use as many sentence patterns as possible in PART III. Alternatively, you may work in pairs on a chosen topic, search the information on the internet, write the introduction and then present it to the class.

_____

_____

_____

PART IV　REFLECTION

Health preservation has been a heated topic in the history of human life. With the development of economy, Chinese people's living standard is improving day by day. A growing number of people choose to engage in physical activities with greater enthusiasm. At the same time, many health promotion programs are broadcast on radio or TV.

Please search the internet for information on **health preservation** and think about the following questions:

1) Why are people becoming enthusiastic about health preservation?

2) What can people do to preserve health?

Unit 7

Overseas Development of Traditional Chinese Medicine

LEARNING OUTCOMES

This unit offers you opportunities to:

- **expound** the challenges that traditional Chinese medicine (TCM) meets during overseas dissemination
- **introduce** the international development of TCM
- **use** the words and expressions related to the overseas development of TCM
- **reflect** on the spread and regulation of TCM in foreign countries

PART I   LISTENING AND SPEAKING

Before you listen

In this section you will hear a short passage entitled "Prescribing Chinese Medicine Illegal in UK Unless Tested". The following words may be of help.

illegal /ɪˈliːg(ə)l/	a.	非法的, 不合法的
preparation /ˌprepəˈreɪʃ(ə)n/	n.	制剂
tablet /ˈtæblɪt/	n.	片剂, 药片
unlicensed /ʌnˈlaɪs(ə)nst/	a.	无执照的, 无资格证的
prohibitive /prə(ʊ)ˈhɪbɪtɪv/	a.	（指价格等）过高的
manufactory /ˌmænjʊˈfækt(ə)ri/	n.	制造厂, 工厂
impose /ɪmˈpəʊz/	vt.	强加, 强迫
clash /klæʃ/	n.	冲突

While you listen

Listen to the passage carefully and fill in each of the blanks marked from 1) to 10) according to what you have heard.

Prescribing Chinese Medicine Illegal in UK Unless Tested

ER-7-1
Listening
practice

In China, Chinese herbal production is a thriving and ancient industry, but it will be illegal in Britain for Chinese doctors to prescribe these preparations unless tested and licensed.

Dr. Han Yu has been a TCM practitioner for thirty years. She has 1) _____ her career in Britain. She says the active 2) _____ make it impossible to catalog Chinese medicine in the same way as the Western counterparts.

Britain's TCM practitioners will be allowed to continue 3) _____ loose herbs like these. The restriction will be set for medicines prescribed in the form of 4) _____ or liquids.

UK medicines 5) _____ agency said: "Natural doesn't always mean safe and some 6) _____ herbal products can be harmful and some may have serious side effects."

Without support of the big producers of prepared medicines in China, however, costs have proven 7) _____.

According to Dr. Han Yu, TCM practitioners in UK lose a lot of 8) _____, because they don't have many things to sell to them.

TCM has important supporters in UK, significantly Health Secretary Jeremy Hunt, but the changes have been 9) _____ by the European Union.

笔记

This is less a 10) _____ of culture than it is a clash of administrators—the European Union and British government depending on tight scientific tests, the Chinese producers of herbal medicines depending on a thousand years of experience.

After you listen

Please discuss with your partner the following questions and give your presentation to the class.

1) Are natural herbs always safe? Please give examples to illustrate your point.

2) What is the attitude of the British government toward the use of Chinese herbal preparations?

笔记

PART II READING

Text A

An Historical Review and Perspective on the Impact of Acupuncture on U.S. Medicine and Society

1　The impact and status of acupuncture in the United States have waxed and waned over the years. In 1997, the National Institutes of Health (NIH)①, after mounting evidence from clinical trials, formally acknowledged acupuncture for its value in relieving pain, nausea after surgery or chemotherapy, and morning sickness;② and effectiveness in treating conditions such as headaches, asthma, stroke rehabilitation and **fibromyalgia**. The NIH also recommended that acupuncture be taught in medical schools.

2　Through the eighteenth, nineteenth, and twentieth centuries, interest in acupuncture within the medical establishment fluctuated. In the early 1800s, articles about acupuncture were published in several U.S. medical journals. Dr. Franklin Baché, a physician, experimented on prisoners (published in the *North American Medical and Surgical Journal*③ in 1826) and concluded that acupuncture was, at the time, the most effective pain management technique. In 1829, a surgical book, *Elements of Operative Surgery*,④ contained a section describing acupuncture techniques, and, in 1836, Dr. William Markley Lee wrote an article in the *Southern Medical Journal*⑤ recommending acupuncture for pain relief. In the same year, he also published, in the *Boston Medical and Surgical Journal*,⑥ an article entitled "Acupuncture as a Remedy for Rheumatism".

3　Unfortunately, this information did not arouse significant interest in the U.S. medical establishment, and acupuncture pretty much faded from American medical scene. Very little about acupuncture was mentioned for almost a quarter of a century until 1859, when Dr. Samuel Gross, in *A System of Surgery*,⑦ discussed acupuncture, saying its advantages had been **overrated**. Although there was some lingering interest in the last half of the eighteenth century, only six articles on acupuncture were published. In 1892, Sir William Osler stated in his classical textbook *The Principles and Practices of Medicine*⑧ that **lumbar** acupuncture is the most efficient treatment for managing acute pain. This same book was republished by D. Appleton and Company in New York, NY, in six editions.

---

① National Institutes of Health (NIH)：美国国立卫生研究院。
② morning sickness: 妊娠呕吐。
③ *North American Medical and Surgical Journal*:《北美医学与外科杂志》。
④ *Elements of Operative Surgery*:《外科手术要素》。
⑤ *Southern Medical Journal*:《南方医学杂志》。
⑥ *Boston Medical and Surgical Journal*:《波士顿医学和外科学杂志》。
⑦ *A System of Surgery*:《外科系统》。
⑧ *The Principles and Practices of Medicine*:《医学原理与实践》。

However, interest in acupuncture remained confined to **sporadic** academic curiosity.

4   Acupuncture remained relatively unknown to the U.S. public until former President Nixon's trip to China in 1972, where acupuncture as a potentially useful medical modality was noticed by the visiting people from the United States. Upon his return, Major General Walter R. Tkach, of the U.S. Air Force and physician to Nixon, wrote an article in the July 1972 issue of *Reader's Digest*,[①] entitled, "I Watched Acupuncture Work,"which helped to popularize acupuncture in the United States. Just prior to Mr. Nixon's trip to China, James Reston, vice president of the *New York Times*, had an **appendectomy** performed in Beijing, China. Under acupuncture anesthesia, he was awake during the entire surgical procedure.

5   Historically, acupuncture anesthesia was first used for dental operations in China, followed by **tonsillectomies**, **thyroidectomies**, **hernia** repairs,[②] and changing of burn **dressings**. In 1972, the first two cases using acupuncture anesthesia/**analgesia** for surgical operations were performed in the United States at the Hospital of Albert Einstein College of Medicine in the Bronx, New York.

6   Today, acupuncture has been used for almost all varieties of surgical procedures. Thousands of open heart operations have been performed under acupuncture, with a success rate of >90%. Even children as young as 10 years old have had congenital heart problems[③] repaired under acupuncture, including **ventricular** and **atrial septal** defects,[④] pulmonary **stenosis**[⑤], and **tetralogy** of Fallot.[⑥] Operations for acquired heart disease have also been performed successfully with acupuncture.

7   There have been various degrees of acceptance and influences on society in general, and the health care system in particular. In the United States, acupuncture anesthesia for surgery is currently rarely done because it is more time consuming and does not achieve the total muscle relaxation that general anesthesia does. Nevertheless, acupuncture has been more widely used since the NIH acknowledged this modality's usefulness. There are many hospitals with acupuncturists on staff. It has been estimated that nearly 20 million Americans have tried acupuncture for various **ailments** and the number of acupuncture procedures almost tripled between 2000 and 2010. According to Yemeng Chen, the president of the New York College of Traditional Chinese Medicine, there are currently 16,000 acupuncturists in the United States (personal communication[⑦]). Throughout professional sports— from football to baseball to tennis and track and field— a growing number of athletes are seeking acupuncture to treat injuries, musculoskeletal tenderness,[⑧] inflammation and pain. Many patients in the United States routinely rely on acupuncture

---

①　*Reader's Digest:*《读者文摘》。

②　hernia repairs: 疝气修补术。

③　congenital heart disease: 先天性心脏病。

④　ventricular and atrial septal defects: 房室隔缺损。

⑤　pulmonary stenosis: 肺动脉瓣狭窄。

⑥　tetralogy of Fallot: 法洛四联症。

⑦　personal communication: 私人通信,私下交流。

⑧　musculoskeletal tenderness: 骨骼肌肉疼痛。

笔记

to alleviate non-sports–related health problems—including allergies, asthma, flu, stress, depression, insomnia, irritable bowel syndrome,① **sciatic** pain,② carpal tunnel syndrome,③ and discomforts from post-cancer therapy.

8   Presently, almost every state in the United States has laws regulating acupuncture practice. There are 55 acupuncture schools in the United States, and many practitioners in this country have received their certificates. Many licensed physicians and dentists acquired their acupuncture licenses through continuing education, and several universities offer acupuncture courses to both post and predoctoral students of health science. In addition, an increasing number of insurance companies cover acupuncture costs for patients. Since 1975, author D.P.L. has offered acupuncture information and instruction to postdoctoral dental residents at Sacred Heart Hospitals and Lehigh Valley Health Network, both in Allentown, PA, and also to predoctoral dental students at University of Pennsylvania since 1994 as part of an elective course on Pain and Anxiety Control. Clinicians seeking continuing education credits and certificates are also offered similar acupuncture courses as part of **intravenous**-sedation④ workshops at St. Joseph Hospital of Seton Hall University School of Health and Medical Sciences.

9   In the United States, both acupuncture and herbal medicine are often practiced as two distinctive entities and disciplines, although both are often combined in China to enhance their therapeutic effects. Acupuncture has been incorporated in many clinical situations, including use for patients who are allergic to local or general anesthetic drugs; patients with psychiatric conditions who are sensitive to the side-effects of conventional medications such as **tranquilizers** and other mood-changing drugs; patients who tolerate opioid analgesics⑤ poorly; and patients with cancer who need high doses of **narcotics** to relieve severe pain. Nevertheless, patients with this pain can benefit from acupuncture treatment, because of the release of β-endorphin,⑥ **serotonin**, **dopamine**, and **norepinephrine** resulting from acupuncture stimulation. Acupuncture has been substituted for those drugs in pain and anxiety management, and can be used in conjunction with conventional medications to reduce drug dosing, so that patients will have fewer side-effects and minimized potential for drug addiction.⑦ Also, acupuncture and moxibustion could also help to correct **breech fetal** position and increase fetal safety as well as reducing the need for Caesarian section.⑧

10   The advantages of acupuncture anesthesia are that the patient remains conscious and able to communicate, has minimal **postoperative** pain, and has fewer side-effects or serious complications. However, the lengthy **induction** needed may **preclude** the routine

---

① irritable bowel syndrome: 肠易激综合征。
② sciatic pain: 坐骨神经痛。
③ carpal tunnel syndrome: 腕管综合征。
④ intravenous-sedation: 静脉镇静。
⑤ opioid analgesics: 阿片类镇静剂。
⑥ β-endorphin: β 内啡肽。
⑦ drug addiction: 药物成瘾。
⑧ caesarian section: 剖宫产术。

笔记

160

use of acupuncture anesthesia in the United States. However, for patients whose airways are difficult to maintain for general anesthesia, acupuncture anesthesia may be the solution to that problem.

11   Acupuncture anesthesia can also benefit medically compromised patients, young children, patients with severe chronic obstructive pulmonary disease or **emphysema**, chronic bronchitis, **acidosis**, severe asthma (bronchial and cardiac), pulmonary edema, **pleurisy**, advanced **tuberculosis**, massive pulmonary **embolism**, severe pneumonia, advanced lung cancer, or pulmonary **fibrosis**.

12   Acupuncture occupies a unique place in modern medicine. Research on acupuncture has taken place in many universities and research institutions around the world, increasing our understanding of how the human body works. Knowledge has been greatly increased especially in the areas of physiology, biochemistry, pharmacology, **kinesiology**, neurology, and **neuroanatomy**. By integrating Eastern and Western medicines, both disciplines can be complementary to each other for the benefit of patients.

Reference: LU D P, LU G P. An historical review and perspective on the impact of acupuncture on U.S. medicine and society [J/OL]. Med Acupunct, 2013, 25 (5):311-316. (2013-10). http://www.ncbi.nlm.nih.gov/pmc/articles/PMC3796320/. DOI:10.1089/acu.2012.0921.

New Words

fibromyalgia /ˌfaɪbrəʊmaɪˈældʒɪə/	*n.*	a rheumatic condition characterized by muscular or musculoskeletal pain with stiffness and localized tenderness at specific points on the body 纤维性肌痛
overrate /ˌəʊvəˈreɪt/	*vt.*	have a higher opinion of (sb. or sth.) than is deserved 高估;评价过高
lumbar /ˈlʌmbə/	*a.*	relating to the lower part of the back 腰部的
sporadic /spəˈrædɪk/	*a.*	occurring at irregular intervals or only in a few places; scattered or isolated 不定时的;零星的
appendectomy /ˌæp(ə)nˈdektəmi/	*n.*	a surgical operation to remove the appendix 阑尾切除术
tonsillectomy /ˌtɒnsɪˈlektəmi/	*n.*	a surgical operation to remove the tonsils 扁桃体切除术
thyroidectomy /ˌθaɪrɔiˈdektəmi/	*n.*	removal of the thyroid gland by surgery 甲状腺切除术
hernia /ˈhəːnɪə/	*n.*	a condition in which part of an organ is displaced and protrudes through the wall of the cavity containing it 疝气

dressing /ˈdresɪŋ/	*n.*	a piece of material used to cover and protect a wound 敷料
analgesia /ˌæn(ə)lˈdʒiːzɪə/	*n.*	the condition of being unable to feel pain while conscious 镇痛
ventricular /venˈtrɪkjʊlə/	*a.*	of or relating to a ventricle（室）of the heart 心室的
atrial /ˈeɪtrɪəl/	*a.*	of or relating to an atrium 心房的
septal /ˈsept(ə)l/	*a.*	relating to a septum or septa 隔膜的，间隔的
stenosis /stɪˈnəʊsɪs/	*n.*	the abnormal narrowing of a passage in the body 狭窄
tetralogy /tɪˈtrælədʒi/	*n.*	a set of four related symptoms or abnormalities frequently occurring together 四联症
ailment /ˈeɪlm(ə)nt/	*n.*	an illness, typically a minor one 疾病，小恙
sciatic /saɪˈætɪk/	*a.*	of or affecting the sciatic nerve; suffering from or liable to sciatica 臀部的；坐骨的；坐骨神经的
intravenous /ˌɪntrəˈviːnəs/	*a.*	existing or taking place within, or administered into, a vein or veins 静脉的，静脉注射的
tranquilizer /ˈtræŋkwɪlaɪzə/	*n.*	a medicinal drug taken to reduce tension or anxiety 镇静剂
narcotic /nɑːˈkɒtɪk/	*n.*	a drug which induces drowsiness, stupor, or insensibility, and relieves pain 麻醉药，镇静剂
serotonin /ˌserəˈtəʊnɪn/	*n.*	a compound present in blood platelets and serum, which constricts the blood vessels and acts as a neurotransmitter 血清素
dopamine /ˈdəʊpəmiːn/	*n.*	a compound present in the body as a neurotransmitter and a precursor of other substances including adrenaline 多巴胺
norepinephrine /ˌnɔːrepɪˈnefrɪːn/	*n.*	a hormone which is released by the adrenal medulla and by the sympathetic nerves and functions as a neurotransmitter 去甲肾上腺素
breech /briːtʃ/	*n.*	(*archaic*) a person's buttocks [古] 臀部
fetal /ˈfiːt(ə)l/	*a.*	relating to a fetus 胎儿的

postoperative /ˌpəʊst'ɒp(ə)rətɪv/	a.	during, relating to, or denoting the period following a surgical operation 手术后的
induction /ɪn'dʌkʃ(ə)n/	n.	the action or process of bringing about or giving rise to sth. 诱发
preclude /prɪ'kluːd/	vt.	prevent from happening; make impossible 妨碍;阻止
emphysema /ˌemfɪ'siːmə/	n.	a condition in which the air sacs of the lungs are damaged and enlarged, causing breathlessness 肺气肿
acidosis /ˌæsɪ'dəʊsɪs/	n.	an excessively acid condition of the body fluids or tissues 酸中毒
pleurisy /'plʊərɪsi/	n.	inflammation of the pleurae, which impairs their lubricating function and causes pain when breathing, causing by pneumonia and other diseases of the chest or abdomen 胸膜炎
tuberculosis /tjʊˌbəːkjʊ'ləʊsɪs/	n.	an infectious bacterial disease characterized by the growth of nodules (tubercles) in the tissues, especially the lungs 肺结核
embolism /'embəlɪz(ə)m/	n.	obstruction of an artery, typically by a clot of blood or an air bubble 栓塞
fibrosis / faɪ'brəʊsɪs/	n.	thc thickening and scarring of connective tissue, usually as a result of injury 纤维化
kinesiology /kɪˌniːsɪ'ɒlədʒi/	n.	the study of the mechanics of body movements 人体运动学
neuroanatomy /ˌnjʊərəʊə'nætəmi/	n.	the anatomy of the nervous system 神经解剖学

Phrases and expressions

wax and wane	起伏,起落,消长
stroke rehabilitation	脑卒中康复
pain management	疼痛治疗
fade from	消退;减退
arouse interest	引发……兴趣
medical modality	治疗方式;医学模式
acupuncture anesthesia/analgesia	针刺麻醉 / 镇痛
dental operation	牙科手术

笔记

on staff	在职;在岗
track and field	田径
continuing education	继续教育
elective course	选修课
therapeutic effect	疗效
high dose	大剂量
conventional medication	常规药物
breech fetal position	胎儿臀位
chronic obstructive pulmonary disease	慢性阻塞性肺疾患
chronic bronchitis	慢性支气管炎
pulmonary edema	肺水肿
advanced tuberculosis	肺结核晚期
massive pulmonary embolism	大面积肺栓塞
pulmonary fibrosis	肺纤维化

Task One　Preview

1. Learn the following roots and affixes. Write out the Chinese meaning of the given words.

Roots/ Affixes	Meaning of roots/affixes	Words	Chinese meaning of the given words
acid	sour	acidity	_____
		acidosis	_____
-algia	pain	arthralgia	_____
		fibromyalgia	_____
append (o)	appendix	appendectomy	_____
		appendicitis	_____
atri (o)	atrium	atrial	_____
		atrioventricular	_____
chem (o)	chemistry	chemotaxis	_____
		chemotherapy	_____
fasci (o)	fibrous band	fascial	_____
		fasciitis	_____
infra-	under, beneath, below	infrasonic	_____
		infrastructure	_____
kyph (o)	hump	kyphosis	_____
		kyphotic	_____

muscul (o)	muscle	muscularity	_____
		musculoskeletal	_____
over-	much	overlap	_____
		overwhelm	_____
pleur (o)	of pleura	pleurisy	_____
		pleuritis	_____
pulmon (o)-	lung	pulmonary	_____
		pulmonology	_____
sciat (o)	sciatic nerve	sciatic	_____
		sciatica	_____
tetra	four	tetracycline	_____
		tetralogy	_____
thyr (o)	pertaining to thyroid	thyroid	_____
		thyroidectomy	_____
ventricul (o)	ventricle	ventricular	_____
		ventriculomegaly	_____

2. Write down the questions you would like to ask or discuss about the text.

_____

_____

_____

Task Two   Speaking

1. Answer the following questions according to the text.

1) What was the attitude of NIH toward acupuncture therapy?

2) What did Dr. Franklin Baché conclude from his experiment on prisoners?

3) Did acupuncture arouse significant interest in the USA before 1900s?

4) What was the turning point of the prevalence of acupuncture in the USA?

5) What conditions is acupuncture employed for?

6) What is the advantage of acupuncture anesthesia?

7) Who are the patients suitable for acupuncture anesthesia?

8) What is the current status of acupuncture?

2. Work in pairs or groups and exchange views on the following passage.

Registration of TCM Practitioners in Australia

In 2012, Australia became the first and the only Western nation that uniformly recognized and regulated TCM practice. For TCM in Australia (and indeed for China itself), this has been a critical game changer. Without the formal recognition of its practitioners, it is very difficult (even illegal in some circumstances) for Western medical doctors to work with them. Without the regulation of practice, there is little formal recognition of TCM, nor the capacity to integrate and incorporate it into the health care

笔记

of Australians. The National Institute of Complementary Medicine (NICM) based at the University of Western Sydney is Australia's lead agency in the research and regulation of TCM. Researchers at the NICM were instrumental in advocating for the regulation of TCM practitioners and they continue to carry out researches on its products and treatments to improve the standard of care and consumer confidence in Australia. The formal review of TCM commenced in 1995, when the NICM staff negotiated with the State governments of New South Wales, Victoria and Queensland to undertake an extensive review of TCM practice in Australia.

The criteria for the national review were very strict, which focused on developing evidence and data for the State governments to determine whether TCM practice needed to be regulated at all. It is important to note that the government does not generally regulate a health care practice because they feel it deserves to be recognized, but rather because they believe if they don't regulate the profession, then the public is at risk to being exposed to unqualified and unscrupulous practitioners.

In brief, based on the data collected by our team over 10 months, it was clear that the practice of TCM presented with prima facie risks that needed to be managed as much as possible. Our recommendation was to introduce practitioner regulation to ensure adequate standards of education and clinical practice. The Victorian government subsequently agreed to lead the way to establish trial regulation of TCM practice in its state.

In those initial years, we developed guidelines for recognizing practitioner's qualifications, standards of practice, and also developed ways of dealing with unqualified practitioners. The trial in Victoria proved successful; however, no other states adopted this model as the health practitioner regulation by Australian Government was due for a major overhaul (彻底检修). Prior to 2008 each state in Australia regulated its own health professionals. That situation still exists in the USA and in Canada where each country has different regulatory laws. In Australia it was decided that health practitioner regulation should be consistent across the whole country and be centrally regulated. Fourteen professions were included and have been regulated by the Australian Health Professional Registration Association (AHPRA). The professions now covered by AHPRA include medicine, nursing, physiotherapy, pharmacy and others, but in particular includes TCM for the first time.

Reference: BENSOUSSAN A, YU U S. Chinese medicine regulation and development in Australia [J]. Journal of Beijing university of traditional Chinese medicine, 2015, 38 (Supp):28-32.

Topic for discussion: Do you think it is important for TCM practitioners to register officially? Why or why not?

Task Three   Vocabulary

1. Match up each word in column A with its appropriate definition from column B.

Column A	Column B
1) sedation	a. a surgery to remove the tonsils
2) tonsillectomy	b. habitual sleeplessness; inability to sleep
3) sporadic	c. existing or taking place within, or administered into, a vein or veins
4) bronchitis	d. a drug which induces drowsiness, stupor, or insensibility, and relieves pain
5) insomnia	e. the action of administering a drug to produce a state of calm or sleep
6) intravenous	f. relating to a fetus
7) narcotic	g. occurring at irregular intervals or only in a few places; scattered or isolated
8) acidosis	h. obstruction of an artery, typically by a clot of blood or an air bubble
9) fetal	i. inflammation of the mucous membrane in the bronchial tubes
10) embolism	j. an excessively acid condition of the body fluids or tissue
11) tenderness	k. the condition of being unable to feel pain while conscious
12) analgesia	l. sensitivity to pain; soreness

2. Fill in the blanks with the words given below. Change the form where necessary.

submit	deliver	legislation	physiology	hearing
consume	supplementary	philosophy	regulate	theory
practitioner	pragmatic	federation	principle	territory

Chinese Medicine in Canada

Canada is a 1) _____ composed of 10 provinces and 3 territories. The main role of Health Canada (a federal department) is to set and administer national principles as well as to 2) _____ food, health and consumer products in order to help Canadians maintain and improve their health. While the provinces and 3) _____ are responsible for delivering health care to the majority of Canadians, authority of 4) _____ for TCM and acupuncture like all of other health profession is under the jurisdiction of the provincial and territorial governments.

It is worthwhile to mention that TCM is a 5) _____ tradition from which acupuncture, herbology, and other primary TCM therapies derive their 6) _____ base and standard of practice. Actually, the BC government established the College of Acupuncturists of British Columbia (CABC) in 1996. Subsequently, through the extensive efforts of visionary pioneers who requested government regulation of TCM and acupuncture, a public 7) _____ was held by the Health Professions Council in 1997 regarding the designation of TCM. After careful study of the 8) _____ and the testimony at the public hearing, the Council believed that it is more appropriate that one college govern both the 9) _____ of TCM and acupuncture. CABC was expanded to the College of Traditional Chinese Medicine Practitioners and Acupuncturists of British Columbia (CTCMA-BC) by the BC government in 1999. BC became the first Canadian province to offer acupuncture treatments as a 10) _____ benefit for its Medical Services Plan premium assistance recipients. Although there are some associations of acupuncture in other provinces and territories in Canada, such as Saskatchewan, Manitoba, Nova Scotia, Prince Edward Island and New Brunswick, TCM and acupuncture have not yet been legislated by the respective governments.

Reference: CAO B Q. Current status and future prospects of acupuncture and traditional Chinese medicine in Canada [J]. Chinese journal of integrative medicine, 2015, 21 (3):166-172.

Task Four　Translation

1. Study the following sentences and pay attention to the underlined parts.

1) Acupuncture pretty much faded from American medical scene. (para. 3)

2) Very little about acupuncture was mentioned for almost a quarter of a century until 1859. (para. 3)

3) Acupuncture remained relatively unknown to the U.S. public until former President Nixon's trip to China in 1972. (para. 4)

4) Thousands of open heart operations have been performed under acupuncture, with a success rate of >90%. (para. 6)

5) It has been estimated that nearly 20 million Americans have tried acupuncture for various ailments. (para. 7)

6) Acupuncture has been incorporated in many clinical situations. (para. 9)

7) Acupuncture occupies a unique place in modern medicine. (para. 12)

2. Translate the following sentences into English.

1) 别仅仅因为你不再是替代医学俱乐部委员而不再积极参加活动。

2) 咖啡因很有名,但植物学里却很少提及它。

3) 药物学家不知道这种神秘药物的组成成分。

4) 一般情况下,对于肺炎旁积液(parapneumonic effusion)的患者,可以通过 B 超或 CT 定位(localization)进行穿刺治疗。

5) 据估计,目前全球抑郁症患者人数多达 1.2 亿。

6) 你的许多建议已被纳入慢性稳定型心绞痛（angina pectoris）的治疗方案中。

7) 中药学在药理学研究中占有重要地位，许多植物药的临床疗效显著。

Text B

The Challenges of Chinese Medicine Education in the UK

1   TCM in the UK can trace its modest beginnings back to the 1970s. Since this time TCM has gradually raised its profile, slowly built its reputation to offer alternative and adjunct treatment[①] to Western medicine. Education and training were initially provided by private schools but have gradually moved into higher education colleges and universities such as Middlesex University. Training and practice requirements vary across Europe; some countries require TCM practitioners to be fully qualified Western doctors, for example in Italy and France; some countries have US-style licensing exams such as Germany and Switzerland; and some countries have professional bodies that **oversee** criteria for qualifications, similar in the UK, Norway, Denmark and Holland. TCM in Europe is used to treat a wide range of conditions, and requests for treatment are almost entirely at the patient's request (i.e., self-referral[②]). Acupuncture is more extensively used and accepted than Chinese herbal medicine, possibly due to Western herbal medicine competing against Chinese herbal medicine. Availability and quality of herbs in Europe, **albeit** improving, remain a challenge. Each European country tends to have a leading professional body and these bodies usually have connections with private health insurers[③] to cover TCM treatment in certain situations.

2   A profile of typical treatments can include: acupuncture and herbs for **infertility** (primarily female) to enhance and support in vitro fertilization[④] cycles; acupuncture to assist in pregnancy, labor and childbirth; acupuncture and tuina to treat musculoskeletal problems, headaches and **migraines**; acupuncture and herbs for depression and insomnia; and qigong in the treatment of Parkinson's disease, etc.

3   The majority of patients who seek TCM present with long term chronic conditions, typically including clinical symptoms associated with obstetric/gynecological, **dermatological**, gastrointestinal, **psychiatric**, stress-related and **allergic** disorders.

4   Within the spectrum of TCM treatments available, acupuncture is increasingly being recognized and accepted as an adjunct to mainstream UK National Health Service treatments, with doctors, physiotherapists and other non-traditional therapists (particularly those that work with long term chronic pain management) enrolling on acupuncture training programs to incorporate TCM into their practice.

---

①　alternative and adjunct treatment: 替代性或辅助性治疗。

②　self-referral: 自我转诊。

③　private health insurer: 私营健康保险公司。

④　in vitro fertilization: 体外受孕。

5　TCM education or training in Europe is variable and not standardized. Courses are delivered by different providers ranging from small private colleges to universities and medical schools. As a consequence, there are no standard **curricula**, learning outcomes or assessment strategies. Teaching materials are locally controlled; however, the following are accepted as leading authors in the area and their texts are often cited as key reference materials (Giovanni Maciocia is **preeminent** in the field of TCM theory; Peter Deadman is the leading name with regards to acupuncture; and Dan Bensky is recognized as having produced the top text books for Chinese herbs and formula). All the above authors closely follow classic TCM theories and extensively overlap with the Chinese State Administration of TCM standard curriculum.

6　There are four universities providing educational programs in the UK, with the primary focus on postgraduate over undergraduate studies. Over recent years there has been a slowing down in **recruitment** to Bachelor of Science studies in TCM, with many universities struggling to secure sufficient student numbers to make a course viable. This downward trend is partly explained by the view that TCM is not perceived as a "first career option".[1] The emerging profile of UK students represents largely two types of students: (1) those who perhaps have already graduated with a primary degree[2] in medicine, nursing, **physiotherapy**, and are seeking to enhance their practice by undertaking a post qualification; or (2) those who have had a personal interest in TCM and wish to change career direction and train as a TCM practitioner full time. Students who fall within the second group, on successful graduation move into being self-employed practitioners working in private clinics.

7　The vast majority of UK courses are **accredited** by the British Acupuncture Council for acupuncture and the European Herbal and Traditional Practitioners Association for herbal medicine. These bodies have helped to raise and maintain very high standards of teaching in the UK.

8　For Middlesex University, the undergraduate and postgraduate Chinese Medicine program was developed in 1996. It was the first degree course in traditional Chinese medicine in the UK and developed in cooperation with Beijing University of Chinese Medicine. Compared with the education of Chinese medicine in China, the program is much more intensive. The reason for this is because students at Middlesex University undertake their training in four years, but in China it is six years. Other significant differences lie in ensuring that UK students are familiar and well versed in the legislation governing their practice, with teaching and clinical placement reflecting how to meet these requirements.

9　As many of the teachers were trained in China, consideration is also given in management of "Western students" expectations, "associated with how Western medical subjects are delivered". Tutor feedback has indicated that students are less familiar with "philosophy" and more focused on "science". Given the emphasis on philosophy within Chinese

① first career option: 首选职业。
② primary degree: 第一学位。

medicine, time is given on the curricula to introduce and explore the importance of philosophy, not only as part of traditional theories, but also in their future practice. A further challenge is related to the names of the herbs or the acupoints. In addition to employing their Latin name, herbs are also discussed using their "pinyin names" adopted by the *European Pharmacopeia*,[①] which is useful and makes the teaching much easier.

10　One of the key components of training is clinical practice and in 2014, Middlesex University invested in the development of its own affiliated university polyclinic called Park Clinic. In addition to offering TCM, the clinic also offers Western herbal medicine and **Ayurvedic** medicine.[②] The clinic offers state of the teaching **facilities** including an onsite dispensary.

11　Students have the opportunity to work alongside their clinical tutors who are all qualified TCM practitioners. The clinic has two classrooms, which are connected to the **consultation** treatment rooms using "web cameras"[③] which facilitate students observing in "real time" live clinical consultations. Clinical tutors or practitioners move between the treatment room and classroom facilitating student questions and learning.

12　In addition to the Park Clinic, the program has its own herbal garden, which is situated, within the grounds of the university. The herbal garden is attended not only by teaching staff, but also by the students during term time, providing "hands on experience" of working with plants in their natural habitat.

13　The structure of the teaching program contains three components: acupuncture, Chinese herbal medicine and basic conventional medicine including anatomy, physiology, pathology and basic pharmacology. Operating since 1996, TCM education and training has successfully been delivered for 18 years with approximately 500 graduates, many of whom have gone on to promote, teach and practice Chinese medicine in the UK and in Europe.

14　Opportunities for research are currently being pursued by TCM staff in collaboration with colleagues within the Department of Mental Health, Social Work and Integrative Medicine.[④] Projects in the areas of mental health, substance misuse, chronic and long term conditions, aging, women's health and digestive health are being conducted. With laboratories in the university, laboratory-based studies[⑤] are also engaged. The university is particularly interested in therapeutic and technological product development and particularly around quality assurance issues in relation to herbal preparation.

15　Statutory regulation and recognition of the many benefits that TCM can offer continue to be a challenge in the UK. Greater emphasis and investment in evidence-based practice must be a priority if such challenges are to be effectively addressed. The UK and Europe need to continue the move to full integration of TCM alongside the offer of Western medicine.

---

①　*European Pharmacopeia*:《欧洲药典》。
②　Ayurvedic medicine: 阿育吠陀医学,印度医学。
③　web cameras: 网络摄像头。
④　Department of Mental Health, Social Work and Integrative Medicine: 精神卫生、社工及融合医学部。
⑤　laboratory-based studies: 基于实验的研究。

This can best be achieved through **collaboration** not only within Europe itself, but also with the support and partnership of countries with stronger tradition and history in TCM.

Reference: CLANCY C, WANG S S, ZHAO K C, et al. The challenges of Chinese medicine education in Europe: a case study from the UK [J]. Journal of Beijing university of traditional Chinese medicine, 2015, 38 (Supp.): 46-49.

New Words

oversee /ˌəʊvəˈsiː/	vt.	supervise (a person or their work), especially in an official capacity 监管, 监督
albeit /ɔːlˈbiːɪt/	conj.	though 尽管, 即使
migraine /ˈmiːgreɪn/	n.	a recurrent throbbing headache that typically affects one side of the head and is often accompanied by nausea and disturbed vision 偏头痛
dermatological /ˌdɜːmətəˈlɒdʒɪk(ə)l/	a.	pertaining to the branch of medicine concerned with the diagnosis and treatment of skin 皮肤病学的
psychiatric /ˌsaɪkɪˈætrɪk/	a.	relating to mental illness or its treatment 精神疾病的
allergic /əˈlɜːdʒɪk/	a.	caused by or relating to an allergy 敏感的, 过敏性的
curriculum /kəˈrɪkjʊləm/	n.	(pl. curricula) the subjects comprising a course of study in a school or college 课程
preeminent /priːˈemɪnənt/	a.	surpassing all others; very distinguished in some way 杰出的, 出色的
recruitment /rɪˈkruːtm(ə)nt/	n.	the action of enlisting new people in the armed forces 补充, 招聘
physiotherapy /ˌfɪzɪə(ʊ)ˈθerəpi/	n.	the treatment of disease, injury, or deformity by physical methods such as massage, heat treatment, and exercise rather than by drugs or surgery 理疗
accredit /əˈkredɪt/	vt.	(of an official body) give authority or sanction to sb. or sth. when recognized standards have been met 认可; 鉴定合格; 委托, 授权
Ayurvedic /ˌɑːjʊəˈveɪdɪk/	a.	related to the traditional Hindu system of medicine, which is based on the idea of balance in bodily systems and uses diet, herbal treatment, and yogic breathing 印度医学的

facility /fə'sɪlɪti/	*n.*	a place, amenity, or piece of equipment provided for a particular purpose 设施，设备
consultation /ˌkɒnsəl'teɪʃ(ə)n/	*n.*	the action or process of formally consulting or discussing 咨询，请教
collaboration /kəˌlæbə'reɪʃn/	*n.*	the action of working with sb. to produce sth. 合作，协作

Phrases and expressions

trace back to	追溯到……
oversee criteria	监督标准
stress-related disorder	压力性疾病，应激性疾病
allergic disorder	过敏性疾病
chronic pain management	慢性疼痛控制
as a consequence	因此
key reference material	主要参考资料
quality assurance	质量保障
statutory regulation	法令规范，法令规则

Task One　Preview

1. Learn the following roots and affixes. Write out the Chinese meaning of the given words.

Roots/ Affixes	Meaning of roots/affixes	Words	Chinese meaning of the given words
ac-	more, again	accelerate	_____
		accompany	_____
adip (o)-	fat	adipocyte	_____
		adiposity	_____
col	with, together	collaboration	_____
		collect	_____
cruit	grow	recruit	_____
		recruitment	_____
curr-	run	currency	_____
		curriculum	_____
fact	do/make	malefaction	_____
		manufacture	_____
granul (o)	granule	granular	_____
		granuloma	_____

笔记

-ion	condition, state	collaboration	_____
		consultation	_____
-ive	related to	integrative	_____
		preventative	_____
labor	labor	collaborate	_____
		elaborate	_____
laryng (o)	throat	laryngopharynx	_____
		laryngoscope	_____
ophthalm (o)	eye	ophthalmology	_____
		ophthalmopathy	_____
migr-	remove	immigrant	_____
		migratory	_____
pod (o)	foot	podocyte	_____
		podiatrist	_____
pub (o)	genital region	pubis	_____
		pubic	_____
under-	below, secondary to	undergraduate	_____
		underpinning	_____
vok	call, voice	equivoke	_____
		provoke	_____
erythr (o)-	red, red cell	erythremia	_____
		erythroblastoma	_____

2. Write down the questions you would like to ask or discuss about the text.

_____

_____

_____

Task Two　Vocabulary

Choose the word or phrase that can best complete the statements.

1) There is substantial scope for improvement in the way the pharmaceutical companies _____ chief executives.

    A. control　　　　　B. supervise　　　　　C. overdue　　　　　D. oversee

2) The New York and the Rome diagnostic _____ for ankylosing spondylitis (强直性脊柱炎, AS) and the clinical history screening test for AS were evaluated in relatives of AS patients and in population control subjects.

    A. paradigm　　　　　B. criteria　　　　　C. credits　　　　　D. rules

3) Unlike most medical conditions, _____ does not incapacitate, nor does it usually cause physical pain or suffering.

    A. fertility　　　　　B. interactivity　　　　　C. disability　　　　　D. infertility

笔记

4) Nearly everybody gets diarrhea once in a while, and it's usually caused by _____ infections.

   A. gastrointestinal   B. cardiovascular   C. rectal   D. urinary

5) A method for achieving diagnostic validity in psychiatric illness is described, consisting of five_____: clinical description, laboratory study, exclusion of other disorders, follow-up study, and family study.

   A. levels   B. phases   C. categories   D. elements

6) Pollen _____ has a remarkable clinical impact all over Europe.

   A. numbness   B. anxiety   C. allergy   D. irritation

7) Rodney Purkiss, a Melbourne doctor, attempted to _____ prosecution for euthanasia to spur test case.

   A. provoke   B. persuade   C. exert   D. promote

8) Blood transfusion depends on availability of donor material, and concerns over supply and safety have spurred development of methods to _____ blood from stem cells.

   A. eliminate   B. transmit   C. manufacture   D. reduce

9) This research might help avoid the _____ issues of harvesting stem cells from embryos.

   A. conscious   B. conceptive   C. ethnic   D. ethical

10) The psychiatric _____ is reported for a large sample of hyperactive children, meeting research diagnostic criteria.

   A. outlook   B. outcome   C. income   D. outline

11) A majority of people _____ the invention of the artemisin to the team of Tu Yoyo.

   A. accredit   B. acquire   C. apply   D. subscribe

12) An emergency department is a medical treatment _____ specializing in the acute care of patients who present without prior appointment, cither by their own means or by that of an ambulance.

   A. plant   B. equipment   C. facility   D. factory

13) The funding committee has set a high _____ on supporting the protocols for the major diseases.

   A. agenda   B. priority   C. urgency   D. standard

14) Patients with obesity might present with _____ changes, such as acanthosis nigricans (黑棘皮病) and skin tags (皮赘).

   A. degenerative   B. dermatological   C. immune   D. deficient

15) The senior researcher intended to discuss the abundance and importance of introduced Chinese herbs in the _____ of South America.

   A. pharmacy   B. pharmacology

   C. pharmacopoeia   D. pharmacologist

Task Three   Translation

Translate the following expressions into English.

1) 引火归原   2) 循证实践

笔记

3) 孕妇晨吐　　　　　　　　4) 先天性心脏病

5) 疝气修补术　　　　　　　6) 肠易激综合征

7) 腕管综合征　　　　　　　8) 坐骨神经痛

9) 剖宫产术　　　　　　　　10) 药物成瘾

11) 腰痛　　　　　　　　　　12) 针刺镇痛

13) 失眠多梦　　　　　　　　14) (将)风险最小化

15) 止痛　　　　　　　　　　16) 止咳化痰

17) 过敏性疾病　　　　　　　18) 大剂量

19) 质量保证　　　　　　　　20) 法令规范

PART III　TRANSLATION AND WRITING

How to Describe the Overseas Development of Traditional Chinese Medicine

The description of the overseas development of traditional Chinese medicine (TCM) usually covers the following details: 1) When did TCM spread to a foreign country?（中医何时传入一个国家？）2) How did TCM initially spread to a foreign country?（中医以什么方式传入外国？）3) How many TCM practitioners, acupuncturists, Chinese pharmacists are there in a foreign country?（这个国家有多少中医师、针灸师、中药师？）4) How many TCM clinics are there in a foreign country?（这个国家有多少中医诊所？）5) Is there any law or regulation on TCM in a foreign country?（这个国家有中医法律法规吗？）6) How is TCM education in a foreign country?（这个国家中医教育的情况怎么样？）7) What is people's attitude towards TCM in a foreign country?（这个国家的民众对中医的态度怎么样？）

The following sentences or expressions are commonly used to describe the overseas development of TCM.

1) Chinese medicine was introduced to Japan with Chinese culture beginning in the 6th century.

早在公元六世纪，中医随着中国文化交流传入日本。

2) TCM was first discussed by U.S. media sources when *New York Times* reporter James Reston returned from a trip to China where he covered President Nixon's visit to Beijing in 1972.

中医首次被美国的媒体报道源于《纽约时报》记者詹姆斯·雷斯顿在其回国后撰写的尼克松总统 1972 年北京之行的报道。

3) There has been unprecedented growth in the field of acupuncture and moxibustion in the U.S. during the past 30 years.

在过去的 30 年里，针灸在美国得到前所未有的发展。

4) 69% of the Korean population has experienced Chinese medicine, and 60%~70% of allopathic doctors in Japan prescribe herbal medicines for their patients.

有 69% 的韩国人体验过中医疗法，日本有 60% 至 70% 采用对抗疗法的医生也为患者开中药。

5) The percentage of traditional medicine doctors in medical facilities (hospitals and clinics) was the highest in Korea, at 15.26%, followed by Chinese mainland, at 12.63%.

医疗机构（包括医院和诊所）里，传统医学的医师所占比例韩国最大，占 15.26%，其次是中国大陆，占 12.63%。

6) The use of acupuncture has become common in Western society, as there are an estimated 15,000 acupuncturists in Europe.

针灸治疗在西方社会变得常见。据估计，欧洲大概有 15,000 名针灸师。

7) In response to the increasing interest of customers, the workforce of TCM and

acupuncture expands fast in the past decade.

随着顾客需求的不断增加,中医和针灸从业人员在过去十年中增长很快。

8) Such transformation of people's attitude and belief has paralleled both good opportunities and stern challenges for TCM.

伴随着人们态度和观念的转变,中医学迎来了良好的机遇和严峻的挑战。

9) This federal campaign of TCM practitioner registration eases some difficulty for Chinese medicine to incorporate into the mainstream health care system in Australia.

联邦政府要求中医师注册的举措为中医融入澳大利亚主流医疗体系排除了一些困难。

10) Australia, since the year of 2012, has become the pioneer Western country which uniformly recognized and regulated Chinese medical practice nationally.

自 2012 年起,澳大利亚成为了第一个对中医师进行全国统一注册和管理的西方国家。

11) As Chinese medicine prevails to the overseas countries, the worldwide interest in its education and training has been on the rise.

随着中医在海外的传播,世界范围内对中医教育和培训的兴趣也随之升温。

12) The academic exchange between these two countries has benefit for both as conjoint efforts will promote Chinese medicine internationally.

两国间的学术交流使双方受益,因为共同的努力可以促进中医国际化。

13) The NIH Consensus report helped acupuncture make significant strides in the Western allopathic medical community as a palliative therapy for a variety of symptoms and conditions.

美国国立卫生研究院共识报告使针灸这一改善多种症状和疾病的姑息疗法大步跻身于西方对抗疗法医学界。

14) More traditionally trained acupuncturists are gaining an interest in and respect for research.

越来越多接受过传统培训的针灸师也开始对研究感兴趣,并尊重研究。

15) The main therapies of traditional medicine were covered, completely or partially, by national health insurance in China, and in some Western society, a few therapies of traditional Chinese tend to be covered by private health insurance too.

中国的国家医疗保险涵盖全部或部分中医治疗费用,西方国家则不同,私人健康保险仅承担很少几种中医治疗费用。

Sample

A Brief Sketch of TCM Development in Australia

Since the late 20th century, the demand for TCM has been growing steadily in developed Western nations. This trend is also reflected in Australia. 1) Chinese immigrants first brought TCM to Australia during the gold-rush days of the 1800s. However, until the 1970s, its use was confined primarily to ethnic Chinese populations. By 1996, there were an estimated 4,500 TCM practitioners in the Australian population, among them

1,500 practitioners were primarily trained in TCM, the remainder incorporating TCM (particularly acupuncture) into their existing practice in professions such as Western medicine, chiropractic, physiotherapy, and nursing. 2) At that time, it was estimated that there were at least 2.8 million consultations with TCM practitioners each year in Australia.

With respect to education, the 1990s also saw an increase in the number of TCM education courses offered in Australia. 3) Currently, seven TCM programs leading to TCM practice qualifications are accredited by the Australian Acupuncture and Chinese Medicine Association, the largest peak professional association for the TCM profession, to provide degree or diploma entry-level training courses for the profession. Of these, three publicly funded Australian universities, including University of Western Sydney, University of Technology, Sydney, and RMIT University, offer degree programs in TCM.

With respect to regulation of TCM, there are two principal government roles: regulation of products (tools of trade) and regulation of practice (practitioner licensing). TCM products have been regulated in Australia since 1989 under the Therapeutic Goods Act 1989. This Act regulates all herbal medicine products for which therapeutic claims are made. Therapeutic claims based on the traditional use of Chinese medicines are permissible, as are higher order therapeutic claims on the basis of sound scientific evidence. 4) Furthermore, toxicological and safety profiles of the herbal ingredients must have been achieved prior to approval for use of these herbal ingredients in any product.

5) While the Commonwealth Government has developed a strong regulatory approach to Chinese medicines, State and Territory Governments, which have jurisdiction over clinical practice, have been fractured in their approach to regulating practitioners. Like any system of medical intervention, TCM carries risks, and without sufficient barriers to entry to the profession, these risks are exacerbated. There has been considerable evidence that self-regulation does not provide sufficient public protection.

Task One   Translation

Translate the underlined parts in the above sample into Chinese.

1) _____

_____

2) _____

_____

3) _____

_____

4) _____

_____

5) _____

_____

Task Two　Writing

Write a 200-word composition, introducing the prevalence of TCM in a country outside China. Try to use as many sentence patterns as possible in PART Ⅲ. Alternatively, you may work in pairs on a chosen topic, search the information on the internet, write the composition and then present it to the class.

_____

_____

_____

PART IV   REFLECTION

Some of the overseas countries or regions have been committed to enhancing health services in their states or regions. Given the possible risks arising from TCM practice, regulations of TCM practitioners are being considered. Regulations are believed to make it possible that registered practitioners have to acquire qualifications and professional trainings, ensuring that the public is adequately protected.

Search the internet for information on **the regulation of TCM** in a foreign country and think about the following questions:

1) Why is TCM legislation considered in that particular country or region?

2) What measures have been taken for the regulation of TCM in that particular country or region?

Unit 8

Medical Ethics

LEARNING OUTCOMES

This unit offers you opportunities to:

- **explain** the scope of responsible practice of traditional Chinese medicine (TCM)
- **compare** the ethical quotations by ancient scholars at home and abroad
- **discuss** the medical ethics for TCM practitioners
- **use** the terms related to medical ethics
- **reflect** on some medical ethical issues

PART I   LISTENING AND SPEAKING

Before you listen

In this section you will hear a short passage entitled "A Good Physician Is Second Best to a Good Prime Minister". The following words and phrases may be of help.

aspirant /əˈspaɪərənt/	n.	有抱负的人
neo-confucianism /ˈnɪːəʊ kənˈfjuːʃənɪzm /	n.	理学
maxim /ˈmæksɪm/	n.	箴言;格言
virtuous /ˈvəːtʃuəs/	a.	品德高的;善良的
benevolent /bəˈnevələnt/	a.	仁慈的
second best to		仅次于

While you listen

Listen to the passage carefully and fill in each of the blanks marked from 1) to 10) according to what you have heard.

A Good Physician Is Second Best to a Good Prime Minister

The saying "being a good physician is only second best to being a prime minister" means an aspirant will strive to be a good physician to save people's lives and keep them healthy if he cannot be a prime minister to 1) _____ the country. In fact, this was an age-old idea. It was first proposed by Fan Zhongyan (989–1052), a famous 2) _____, thinker and writer of the Northern Song Dynasty (960–127).

ER-8-1
Listening
practice

Fan was then the vice prime minister of the Northern Song Dynasty and a 3) _____ of the Neo-confucianism. He wrote in his essay *On Yueyang Tower* a maxim: "Be the first to bear hardships before everybody else and the last to 4) _____," which is known to every household. It can be regarded as the declaration of the 5) _____ of Chinese scholar-officials.

Fan was deeply influenced by Mencius' thought of enjoying happiness with people. Before he 6) _____ of vice prime minister, he expressed that a scholar cherished the hope of having a virtuous emperor who implemented 7) _____ ruling. But only a prime minister could help the common people. If one could not be a prime minister but still wanted to 8) _____ the society and people, there was no better profession than practicing medicine.

Fan regarded being a good prime minister and being a good physician as the ideal 9) _____ of a great man, because they both wanted to help the common people, which was the spirit of a great man 10) _____ by Mencius.

After you listen

Please discuss with your partner the following questions and give your presentation to the class.

1) Please comment on the saying: "Be the first to bear hardships before everybody else and the last to enjoy comforts." What do you think you could do to help others?

2) What qualities do you think a good doctor should have?

PART II   READING

Text A

Scope of Responsible Practice for Traditional Chinese Medicine

1   It is essential that practitioners maintain and actively promote the integrity of traditional Chinese medicine (TCM) and be **scrupulous** in evaluating any diagnostic or therapeutic approach which is not an authentic part of TCM that might be incorporated into a TCM practice.

2   Many practitioners in the West have quickly added to their TCM practice both diagnostic and therapeutic methods that have these characteristics: they have no basis in TCM; they have no support in modern medicine (the accepted medical system in the Western culture); and they can **taint** the field of TCM for all practitioners.

3   One of the primary attractions of TCM is that it has a long history of use, that it has been and continues to be extensively used in its country of origin, and that its component parts are unified by a relatively consistent **dogma**. Patients going to practitioners of Chinese medicine have a reasonable expectation of being provided authentic TCM services, reflecting the best and safest practices from China (or, under the heading Oriental medicine, from Japan, Korea, and other countries that adopted Chinese medical concepts and practices). Chinese medicine is recognized as being a system that, like other health care systems, is liable to be adversely affected by deception, **quackery**, practice by untrained people, and similar problems whereby patients might be exploited by practitioners either willfully or without realizing it (even with best of intentions). TCM literature refers to many instances where these problems arose in China. Patients going to practitioners who are licensed by their respective State governments have a reasonable expectation that such **fraudulent** and non-authentic or amateur practices have been **weeded** out via the required educational process, the testing and licensing processes, and monitoring of practitioners once they have set up their medical business. However, there are **defects** in the current system that allow practitioners to ignore their scope of practice and incorporate techniques not consistent with authentic TCM and not consistent with the high standards of education and monitoring that are expected.

4   Patients can reasonably expect that practitioners of TCM have undergone **rigorous**, prolonged training and appropriate **internship** in order to understand their field of expertise and carry out its techniques with adequate knowledge and skill. Practitioners usually graduate from accredited schools, work (while being students) in professionally supervised clinics, and meet requirements for competence and understanding that are to be maintained and expanded through approved continuing education, as established by state and national organizations. Unfortunately, when adding other techniques to the practice

of TCM, a practitioner might receive little training and the training might be provided by a person who would not meet qualifications consistent with accreditation of schools; the techniques may be ones that are not acceptable within the approved programs or in accordance with their standards, or the board responsible for monitoring and approving such courses may fail to do its important duty of careful oversight. Practitioners and their patients will not have a means for evaluating the training that is received nor the level of competence gained in use of these methods.

5   TCM is regarded, by most practitioners and educators in the field, as a system of great depth, one which requires years of effort to master, far beyond the basics learned in a college program. By adopting non-TCM approaches into the clinical work, the practitioner may be **diverted** from further investigation of his/her field of expertise and licensing, particularly if the adopted methods are **proclaimed** (usually without proof) to resolve difficulties of practice that would otherwise require much study and effort. The problem is compounded when practitioners adopt non-TCM methods soon after completing their basic training, before getting a depth of knowledge and experience from working with TCM; because of limited experience, they may not be able to distinguish between authentic TCM and other methods that are popular **fads**.

6   That these basic issues are not new and not unique to the Western situation can be illustrated by quoting from Qing Dynasty authors. Huai Yuan wrote a warning to physicians of his day, in a book dating from 1808:

> *In medical practice one cannot act at one's own **discretion**. Patients **entrust** physicians with the decision over their life and their death... [the physician] searches for the causes and considers the consequences. He knows the normal and understands the changes... A physician plans in detail and thinks comprehensively. He observes a disease and takes precautions against it to avoid a second. He is glad over a success and yet he is aware that one cannot **repose** on this...Those, however, who surrender to fashionable trends do not carry out their practice **conscientiously**. They place themselves in the greatest light and make use of the need of others in order to **appropriate** their material goods to themselves... A physician has to love and respect himself; only then will he, when he faces a grave disease, possess enough trust in himself. I have studied at great length and in any diagnosis of a disease, I proceed with **exactitude** and conscientiousness; how could I carelessly **acquit** myself of that which others have entrusted to me and which I have promised to them? ... Every patient has to consider the practicing physician a trustworthy person. A physician may examine the respectable [methods] without any further consideration. Yet, if he meets with the **disreputable**, he is first to assure himself of all the details related to it before making a decision.*

7   Xu Dachun, (writing 50 years earlier, in 1757), also warned physicians about the ease

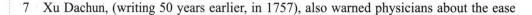

of deceiving patients with wrong ideas:

> *The fact is that patients are people who do not know anything about medicine... When the patients meet someone who knows a little about medical principles, and [who] offers clear-cut discourse and discussion, they will believe what they hear, especially if he displays extraordinary concern and if emotions and face are involved. Who knows that this talk is based on superficial reading and stands for nothing but gossip? Before the people offering [these things] have considered what will happen to the patients following their advice, the patients will have already followed them... As a result, they **recklessly** treat people's illnesses and if these illnesses heal, they consider this their own achievement. If the patient dies, they have done no wrong. They cling only more strongly to their one-sided views... they go on and write books and establish **doctrines** of their own, and thusly **bequeath** harm even to later generations. There are so many such people—one cannot count them.*

8   Although Xu mentions the extreme case of a person dying, which is usually not the situation in modern times, he gives a good analysis; it is easy for a person to claim credit for any improvements that a patient has, and to disregard failures: in the modern situation, a patient doesn't die but simply decides not to come back for another treatment; the practitioner doesn't *see* a failure because of keeping awareness only of those who come back again and again.

9   Huai, Xu, and other Chinese **commentators** were aware that many practitioners of TCM could easily be distracted from their medicine by **promulgators** of disreputable techniques and from hearing presentations by **charismatic** speakers. They worried about people doing superficial investigations and introducing methods that were based on gossip and emotion-based claims. The same can and does happen in the modern world. Practitioners of TCM in the West are particularly susceptible because they are working within a culture that is not **inherently** supportive of their efforts, where the medicine they are licensed to practice is already considered an alternative to what is widely accepted. As a result, the ethical barrier to invasive, superficial, and distracting ideas, a valuable barrier that should exist, is sometimes left too **porous** or removed altogether. The requirement for an ethical barrier is not a matter of having a closed mind, but rather a matter of maintaining appropriate and necessary ethical restrictions under difficult circumstances.

10   It is essential that practitioners of Chinese medicine give *serious* consideration to the introduction of non-TCM techniques into their practice before including them. Schools of Chinese medicine and teachers in the field need to explicitly define what constitutes TCM and emphasize that it has characteristics which patients expect to encounter, including authenticity of the technique as part of TCM, training of the practitioner in the techniques they apply within the accredited courses, and reasonable interpretation of the

scope of practice. The method for evaluating claims of effectiveness and evaluating patient responses to treatments need to become part of the TCM curriculum.

Reference: DHARMANANDA S. Ethics in modern practice of traditional Chinese medicine (TCM) [EB/OL]. (2015-09-20). http://www.itmonline.org/articles/ethics/ethics.htm.

New words

scrupulous /ˈskruːpjʊləs/	a.	(of a person or process) careful, thorough, and extremely attentive to details 严谨的；小心的
taint /teɪnt/	vt.	affect with a bad or undesirable quality 使变质；败坏；玷污
dogma /ˈdɒgmə/	n.	a principle or set of principles laid down by an authority as incontrovertibly true 教义，教条，信条
quackery /ˈkwækəri/	n.	dishonest practices and claims to have special knowledge and skill in some field, typically medicine 庸医的医术
fraudulent /ˈfrɔːdjʊl(ə)nt/	a.	obtained, done by, or involving deception, especially criminal deception 欺骗的，不诚实的；奸诈的
weed /wiːd/	vt.	remove an inferior or unwanted component of a group or collection 消除
defect /ˈdiːfekt/	n.	a shortcoming, imperfection, or lack 瑕疵；欠缺，缺点
rigorous /ˈrɪg(ə)rəs/	a.	extremely thorough and careful 严密的；缜密的；严格的
internship /ˈɪntəːnʃɪp/	n.	the position of a student or trainee who works in an organization, sometimes without pay, in order to gain work experience or satisfy requirements for a qualification（美）实习医师，实习医师期
divert /daiˈvəːt/	vt.	cause sb. or sth. to change course or turn from one direction to another 使……改道，转向
proclaim /prəˈkleɪm/	vt.	announce officially or publicly（正式）宣布，（公开）声明
fad /fæd/	n.	an intense and widely shared enthusiasm for sth., especially one that is short-lived; a craze 一时的流行；一时的风尚

discretion /dɪˈskreʃ(ə)n/	n.	the quality of behaving or speaking in such a way as to avoid causing offence or revealing confidential information 慎重；考虑周到；判断力，辨别力
entrust /ɪnˈtrʌst/	vt.	assign the responsibility for doing sth. to sb. 委托，托付
repose /rɪˈpəuz/	vt.	(literary) lay sth. to rest in or on ［书面语］将……寄托于，安放在……
conscientiously /ˌkɒnʃɪˈenʃəsli/	ad.	in a way that is motivated by one's moral sense of right and wrong 凭良心地；认真负责地
appropriate /əˈprəuprɪeɪt/	vt.	take (sth.) for one's own use, typically without the owner's permission 盗用；侵吞
exactitude /ɪgˈzæktɪtjuːd/	n.	the quality of being exact 正确；严谨
acquit /əˈkwɪt/	vt.	discharge (a duty or responsibility) 除去责任或义务
disreputable /dɪsˈrepjutəb(ə)l/	a.	not considered to be respectable in character or appearance 名誉不好的，不体面的
recklessly /ˈreklɪsli/	ad.	without regard to the danger or the consequences of one's actions; rashly 不在乎地，不顾一切地
bequeath /bɪˈkwiːð/	vt.	pass sth. on or leave sth. to sb. else 将（财物等）遗赠给；将（知识等）传给（后人）
commentator /ˈkɒmənteɪtə/	n.	a person who comments on events or on a text 注解者；评论员
promulgator /ˈprɒm(ə)lgeɪtə/	n.	a person who promotes or makes widely known (an idea or cause) 颁布者，公布者
charismatic /ˌkærɪzˈmætɪk/	a.	exercising a compelling charm which inspires devotion in others 有魅力的；神授的
inherently /ɪnˈhɪərəntli/	ad.	in a permanent, essential, or characteristic way 天性地，固有地
porous /ˈpɔːrəs/	a.	(of a rock or other material) having minute interstices through which liquid or air may pass 能穿透的，能渗透的；有毛孔或气孔的

笔记

189

Phrases and expressions

be incorporated into	合并到……, 被整合到……
have no basis in	在某方面没有（理论）基础
in the country of origin	在起（发）源国家
under the heading of	以……为标题
be liable to	易于……
even with best of intentions	即使出于最好的目的
refer to	指的是……；提到
be consistent with	与……一致的，和谐的
in professionally supervised clinics	在有专业人员指导的诊所
approved continuing education	经过认证的继续教育
in accordance with the standards	符合标准
a system of great depth	深奥的体系
far beyond the basics learned in a college program	远远超出大学课程中学到的基础知识
be diverted from	使分心
without proof	没有依据，没有证据
get a depth of knowledge	深入了解（获得）知识
be unique to	属于特定（人或者地方）的，具有特定风格的
at one's own discretion	依据，随某人的意愿处理
take precautions against	对……采取预防措施
acquit oneself of	宣告某人无罪；原谅某人
be inherently supportive of	从本质（根本）上支持
within the accredited courses	在认可（学分）的课程之内
the scope of TCM practice	中医行医范围

Task One　Preview

1. Learn the following roots and affixes. Write out the Chinese meaning of the given words.

Roots/ Affixes	Meaning of roots/affixes	Words	Chinese meaning of the given words
-ase	enzyme	maltase	_____
		transaminase	_____
brady-	slow	bradycardia	_____
		bradypepsia	_____

calc (o)/	calcium	hypercalcemia	_____
calci (o)		calcification	_____
esthes/	sense	anesthesia	_____
esthesi (o)		esthesioneurosis	_____
clast	to break, destroy	osteoclast	_____
		osteoclastoma	_____
cyt (o)/cyte	cell	cytobiology	_____
		monocyte	_____
dent (o)	teeth	dentalgia	_____
		dentistry	_____
enter (o)	small intestine	enteritis	_____
		enteropathy	_____
gloss (o)	tongue	glossalgia	_____
		glossopharyngeal	_____
-lalia	indicating a speech	dyslalia	_____
	defect or abnormality	glossolalia	_____
odont	teeth	odontogenesis	_____
		periodontitis	_____
-oid	-like, like that of	carotenoid	_____
		rheumatoid	_____
or (o)	mouth	orolingual	_____
		peroral	_____
-pepsia/-peps	digestion	dyspepsia	_____
		pepsic	_____
-phasia	speech	aphasia	_____
		monophasia	_____
splen (o)	spleen	splenocyte	_____
		splenomegaly	_____
stomat (o)	mouth	enterostomy	_____
		stomatology	_____
tachy-	fast	tachycardia	_____
		tachypnea	_____

2. Write down the questions you would like to ask or discuss about the text.

_____

_____

_____

191

Task Two　Speaking

1. Answer the following questions according to the text.

1) Why should TCM practitioners maintain the integrity of traditional Chinese medicine?

2) What do people expect when going to TCM practitioners?

3) What are some of the bad phenomena, and attractions of TCM practice in the Western world?

4) What is the negative consequence of adopting non-TCM approaches into TCM clinical work?

5) What is the main idea of Huai Yuan's quotation?

6) What is the main idea of Xu Dachun's quotation?

7) What is TCM regarded as in Western society?

8) Why should an ethical barrier be set in Western society for TCM practitioners?

2. Work in pairs or groups and exchange views on the quotation in the following excerpt.

It is vital that persons who offer professional services in the field of TCM maintain adequate knowledge of all the relevant subjects in order to give a level of service consistent with the current state of the art. Xu Dachun, about 250 years ago, commented on the need for physicians to continually study:

Today's physicians possess no skills. They do not read a single book. Hence those who merely browse through the medical literature [become prevalent]... Those browsers believe themselves to be increasingly right after some time. [Yet], in the beginning they harm other people through mistaken treatments; then they harm their relatives through their mistaken treatments; in the end, they harm themselves through mistaken treatments.

Physicians whose training is insufficient may still avoid harming people as long as they are able to follow proper principles. And if they are able to remain modest, and if they attach great importance to studying, their knowledge will progress every day, and each of their therapies will result in a cure. Hence their fame and reputation will increase and many people will seek their help as a consequence— with riches following them. If one searches for nothing but riches, one will miss both fame and riches. Why do the physicians increase their own problems by neglecting one [studying] and going for the other [seeking rewards]?

Reference: UNSCHULD P U. Forgotten traditions of ancient Chinese medicin [M]. Brookline, MA: Paradigm Publications, 1990.

Topic for discussion: What do you learn from the above quotation?

Task Three   Vocabulary

1. Match up each word in Column A with its appropriate definition from Column B.

Column A	Column B
1) internship	a. a shortcoming, imperfection, or lack
2) scrupulous	b. expert skill or knowledge in a particular field
3) doctrine	c. affect with a bad or undesirable quality
4) authentic	d. the quality of being exact
5) entrust	e. the act of granting credit or recognition
6) taint	f. in a permanent, essential, or characteristic way
7) defect	g. a belief or set of beliefs held and taught by a Church, political party
8) expertise	h. a student or trainee who works in an organization in order to gain work experience or satisfy requirements for a qualification
9) accreditation	i. genuine; of undisputed origin and not a copy
10) exactitude	j. assign the responsibility for doing sth. to sb.
11) bequeath	k. (of a person or process) careful, thorough, and extremely attentive to details
12) inherently	l. pass sth. on or leave sth. to sb. else

2. Fill in the blanks with the words given below. Change the form where necessary.

improve	increase	ill	personal	progress
regard	slow	diagnose	present	content
medicine	exist	formulate	develop	title

Ancient Chinese Medical Ethics

The seventh century saw the maturity of medical ethics in ancient China, embodied in two special chapters regarding the requirements for a doctor in the book *Qianjin Fang* (*Prescriptions Worth a Thousand Pieces of Gold*) written by the famous physician Sun Simiao (581-682). The 1) _____ of the two chapters are "Perfect Proficiency of a Great Doctor" and "Practicing and Conducts of a Great Doctor", respectively. These 2) _____ the standards for ancient traditional medical ethics, including:

• Be erudite (博学的) in 3) _____ knowledge and diligent in learning. All doctors should progress constantly and keep 4) _____ their skill of the medical art and technical know-how.

• Be sympathetic to patients and serve them wholeheartedly. Serve all patients equally, 5) _____ of their age, sex, wealth, rank, nationality and intelligence. Treat all patients as if they were your own relatives and their 6) _____ as if it were your own suffering. Meet the patient at any time or any place when a doctor's help is needed, notwithstanding any danger.

- Be painstakingly careful in 7) _____ a disease. Think carefully when prescribing treatment. Be objective and avoid any personal considerations of responsibility or being swayed by personal feelings.

- Be solemn in one's conduct without making any 8) _____ demands: no humor, demands for money, or sexual issues should be raised.

- Be respectful to one's tutor and profession. Avoid any arrogance and rashness. Do not criticize other doctors' skill or conduct in the 9) _____ of a patient. Do not be arrogant about one's own achievement. Learn from other doctors to ensure one's own 10) _____, only charlatans（骗子，冒充内行者）are jealous of other doctor's superb skills.

Task Four Translation

1. Study the following sentences and pay attention to the underlined parts.

1) It is essential that practitioners maintain and actively promote the integrity of Chinese medicine and be scrupulous in evaluating any diagnostic or therapeutic approach which is not an authentic part of TCM that might be incorporated into a TCM practice. (para. 1)

2) Patients going to practitioners of Chinese medicine have a reasonable expectation of being provided authentic TCM services, reflecting the best and safest practices from China. (para. 3)

3) However, there are defects in the current system that allow practitioners to ignore their scope of practice and incorporate techniques not consistent with authentic TCM and not consistent with the high standards of education and monitoring that are expected. (para.3)

4) TCM is regarded, by most practitioners and educators in the field, as a system of great depth, one which requires years of effort to master, far beyond the basics learned in a college program. (para. 5)

5) A physician has to love and respect himself; only then will he, when he faces a grave disease, possess enough trust in himself. (para. 6)

6) The requirement for an ethical barrier is not a matter of having a closed mind, but rather a matter of maintaining appropriate and necessary ethical restrictions under difficult circumstances. (para. 9)

7) It is essential that practitioners of Chinese medicine give serious consideration to the introduction of non-TCM techniques into their practice before including them. (para. 10)

2. Translate the following sentences into English.

1) 中医有着与西医不同的思想体系，认识到这一点非常重要。

2) 他们对中医在美国的发展寄予了很高的期望。

3) 强迫医生向患者提供不准确的信息是不符合医学伦理的。

4) 许多西方人对中医了解不多,其实中医在中国使用历史和范围远远超出他们所了解的中医概念。

5) 在古代中国,中医师在独立行医之前必须跟着师父当学徒多年,学习中医诊断和治疗方法以及中草药知识。唯有如此,他才可能得到师父允许开馆行医。

6) 医生不能明确诊断、解释和/或治疗、治愈慢性背痛患者似乎不是解救了患者,而是延长了患者对医生的依赖。

7) 风险评估很少考虑对婴儿和儿童的潜在健康影响。

Text B

Traditional Chinese Medicine Practitioners' Ethical Code and Relationships with Patients

1　Traditional Chinese medicine (TCM) practitioners have, since ancient times, been respected and trusted by the people in their practice of TCM. They are looked upon for the relief of suffering and ailments. With the trust reposed in them, TCM practitioners must do their best to maintain a high level of self-discipline, competence, and standard of professional conduct and provide professional, proper and adequate service in their prescribed practice of TCM.

2　While the profession must adhere to the laws governing society and its practice, it must also be self-regulating, as society at large may not have the necessary knowledge or the experience of medical practice to make determinations on professional matters. This self-regulation must be vigorously and fairly pursued so that the profession continues to enjoy the trust of the society. TCM practitioners are **exhorted** to keep the following ethical code firmly in mind in the course of their practice.

TCM practitioners' ethical code

3　Patients and the public must be able to trust TCM practitioners **implicitly** with their lives and well-being. To justify this trust, TCM practitioners have to maintain a good standard of care, conduct and behavior. The Traditional Chinese Medicine Practitioners Board prescribes an "Ethical Code" which TCM practitioners are expected to uphold. These principles are applicable to a wide variety of circumstances and situations. **Adherence** to the Code will enable the public at large to have trust and confidence in the profession.

4　TCM practitioners must use the Code as a **yardstick** for their own conduct and behavior. In addition, it is advisable for TCM practitioners to understand medical ethics, train in ethical analysis and decision making, develop knowledge, skills and attitude needed to deal with ethical conflicts. Consult with colleagues, ethical committees and other experts when

笔记

ethical conflicts arise.

5   In general, a TCM practitioner is expected to:

- Be dedicated to providing competent, **compassionate** and appropriate medical care to patients.

- Be an **advocate** for patients' care and well-being and endeavor to ensure that patients suffer no harm.

- Provide access to and treat patients without prejudice of race, religion, **creed**, social standing, disability or financial status. A TCM practitioner shall also be prepared to treat patients on an emergency or **humanitarian** basis when circumstances permit.

- Abide by all laws and regulations governing TCM practice and abide by the "Ethical Code" of the TCM profession.

- Maintain the highest standards of moral integrity and intellectual honesty.

- Treat patients with honesty, dignity, respect and consideration, **upholding** their right to be adequately informed and their right to self-determination.

- Maintain a professional relationship with patients and their relatives and not abuse this relationship through inappropriate personal relationships or for personal gain.

- Keep confidential all medical information about patients.

- Regard all fellow professionals as colleagues, treat them with dignity, accord them respect and manage those under his/her supervision with **professionalism**, care and **nurturing**.

- Be open, truthful, factual and professionally modest in communications with other members of the profession, with patients and with the public at large.

- Maintain professionalism in informing the public about his/her services, ensuring that information projected is purely factual and **devoid** of any attempt at self-**aggrandizement**.

- Keep **abreast** of TCM knowledge relevant to practice and ensure that clinical and technical skills are maintained.

- Participate in activities contributing to the good of the community, including public health education.

- Endeavour to abide by the "Ethical Code" when making use of modern or new technology in treatment modalities, communication means or information handling.

The Code shall be applied to clinical practice and all areas of professional activity conducted by TCM practitioners.

TCM practitioners' relationshssips with patients

6   The TCM practitioners should follow the following guidelines when dealing with patients. Firstly, patients shall be treated with **courtesy**, consideration, compassion and respect. They shall also be offered the right to **privacy** and dignity. It is recommended that a female **chaperone** be present where a male TCM practitioner examines a female patient. This will protect both the patient's right to privacy and dignity, as well as the TCM practitioner from complaints of **molestation** or other **allegations** of **outrage** of modesty. On the other hand, a TCM practitioner is not obliged to allow himself to be subjected to abuse of any kind by patients or their relatives. Where such abuse occurs, provided that there is no need

for self-defense against physical harm, TCM practitioners shall not **retaliate**, but end the engagement with the patient as quickly as possible, in a professional manner.

7　Secondly, it is a TCM practitioner's responsibility to ensure that a patient under his care is adequately informed about his medical condition and options for treatment so that he is able to participate in decisions about his treatment. If a procedure needs to be performed, e.g. acupuncture, the patient shall be made aware of the benefits, risks and possible complications of the procedure and any alternatives available to him. If the patient is a minor, or of diminished ability to give consent, this information shall be explained to his parent, guardian or person responsible for him for the purpose of his consent on behalf of the patient.

8　Thirdly, a TCM practitioner shall respect the principle of medical **confidentiality** and not disclose without a patient's consent, information obtained in confidence or in the course of attending to the patient. However, confidentiality is not absolute. It may be over-ridden by **legislation**, court orders or when the public interest demands disclosure of such information. An example is national disease registries which operate under a strict framework which safeguards medical confidentiality. There may be other circumstances in which a TCM practitioner decides to disclose confidential information without a patient's consent. When he does this, he must be prepared to explain and justify his decision if asked to do so. A TCM practitioner is expected to take steps to ensure that the means by which he communicates or stores confidential medical information about patients are secure and the information is not accessible to **unauthorized** persons. This is particularly relevant to sending or storing medical information by electronic means, via a website or by email.

9　Fourthly, a TCM practitioner shall provide adequate information to a patient so that he can make informed choices about his further medical management. A TCM practitioner shall provide information to the best of his ability, communicate clearly and in a language that is understood by the patient. A TCM practitioner shall respect a patient's choice of accepting or rejecting advice/treatment that is offered, after steps have been taken to ensure that there is no language barrier and the patient understands the consequences of his choice. He shall also **facilitate** a patient obtaining a second opinion if he so desires.

10　There may be instances of a patient's relatives asking that the patient not be told that he has a fatal or socially embarrassing disease. A TCM practitioner may not withhold this information from the patient unless the TCM practitioner determines that this is in the best interest of the patient. TCM practitioners shall recognize the role of the family in the decision about whether to disclose a diagnosis to a patient and address their concerns adequately.

Reference: Traditional Chinese Medicine Practitioners Board, Singapore. Ethical Code and Ethical Guidelines for TCM Practitioners [EB/OL]. (2006-01).[2015-09-21].

http://www.healthprofessionals.gov.sg/content/dam/hprof/tcmpb/docs/Form_Download/Ethical%20 Code%20and%20Ethical%20Guidelines%20for%20TCMP_E_C.pdf.

New words

exhort /ɪgˈzɔːt/	vt.	strongly encourage or urge sb. to do sth. 劝告，劝说；倡导
implicitly /ɪmˈplɪsɪtli/	ad.	with no qualification or question, absolutely 无条件地，绝对地，无疑问地
adherence /ədˈhɪərəns/	n.	attachment or commitment to a person, cause, or belief 依附；坚持；忠诚
yardstick /ˈjɑːdstɪk/	n.	a standard used for comparison 码尺；尺度
compassionate /kəmˈpæʃ(ə)nət/	a.	feeling or showing sympathy and concern for others 有同情心的；表示怜悯的
advocate /ˈædvəkət/	n.	a person who publicly supports or recommends a particular cause or policy 提倡者，拥护者
creed /kriːd/	n.	a system of religious belief; a faith（尤指宗教）信条，教义；纲领
humanitarian /hjuˌmænɪˈteːrɪən/	a.	concerned with or seeking to promote human welfare 人道主义的；博爱的
	n.	a person who seeks to promote human welfare 人道主义者；博爱主义者
uphold /ʌpˈhəʊld/	vt.	confirm or support (sth. which has been questioned) 支持；赞成；支撑
professionalism /prəˈfeʃ(ə)n(ə)lɪz(ə)m/	n.	the competence or skill expected of a professional 职业水准或特性
nurture /ˈnɜːtʃə/	vt.	care for and protect sb. or sth. while they are growing 养育；培育
devoid /dɪˈvɔɪd/	a.	entirely lacking or free from 缺乏，没有
aggrandize /əˈɡrændaɪz/	vt.	increase the power, status, or wealth of 增大，强化，扩大
abreast /əˈbrest/	ad.	side by side and facing the same way, (usually *abreast of*) alongside or level with sth. 并排地
courtesy /ˈkɜːtɪsi/	n.	the showing of politeness in one's attitude and behaviour towards others 谦恭有礼，礼貌
privacy /ˈprɪvəsi/	n.	a state in which one is not observed or disturbed by other people 隐私，不受公众干扰的状态

chaperone /'ʃæpərəun/	n.	a person who accompanies and looks after another person or group of people 保护人；监护人
molestation /ˌməule'steɪʃ(ə)n/	n.	sexual assault or abuse of a person, especially a woman or child 骚扰
allegation /ˌælɪ'geɪʃ(ə)n/	n.	a claim or assertion that sb. has done sth. illegal or wrong, typically one made without proof 陈述，主张；指控
outrage /'autreɪdʒ/	n.	an extremely strong reaction of anger, shock, or indignation 义愤；愤慨
retaliate /rɪ'tælɪeɪt/	vi.	make an attack in return for a similar attack 报复，反击
confidentiality /ˌkɔnfɪˌdenʃɪ'ælɪti/	n.	the state of keeping or being kept secret or private 机密性
legislation /ˌledʒɪs'leɪʃ(ə)n/	n.	the process of making or enacting laws 立法，制定法律
unauthorized /ʌn'ɔ:θəraɪzd/	a.	not having official permission or approval 未经授权的；未经许可的
facilitate /fə'sɪlɪteɪt/	vt.	make (an action or process) easy or easier 促进，助长；帮助

Phrases and expressions

ethical code	道德准则
adhere to the laws	遵循法律
at large	整体上，总体上
enjoy the trust of the society	得到社会的信任
keep firmly the ethical code in mind	将道德准则牢记在心
in the course of their practice	在行医过程中
have trust and confidence in the TCM profession	对中医专业建立信任和信心
deal with ethical conflicts	处理伦理冲突
ethical committee	伦理委员会
be dedicated to + v-ing/sth.	致力于……
without prejudice of race	没有种族偏见
on humanitarian basis	基于人道主义精神
laws and regulations governing TCM practice	中医医疗行业的法规和条例
abide by the ethical code of the TCM profession	遵守中医行业的道德准则

the right to be informed	知情权
for personal gain	为了（谋取）个人利益
keep confidential all medical information	保守医疗信息秘密
keep abreast of	跟上
the right to privacy and dignity	隐私权和尊严
in a professional manner	以专业的方式
without the patient's consent	未经患者同意
in confidence	私下
a socially embarrassing disease	尴尬难言的疾病

Task One   Preview

1. Learn the following roots and affixes. Write out the Chinese meaning of the given words.

Roots/ Affixes	Meaning of roots/affixes	Words	Chinese meaning of the given words
-ary	pertaining to	extraordinary	_____
		voluntary	_____
bi-/di-	two, double	biceps	_____
		dioxide	_____
hex-	six	hexachromic	_____
		hexadactyly	_____
leuk (o)	white	leukemia	_____
		leukocyte	_____
malacia	abnormal softening	arteriomalacia	_____
		osteomalacia	_____
-penia	decreasing, lack of	cytopenia	_____
		leukocytopenia	_____
pent-	five	pentacyclic	_____
		pentoxide	_____
phage/phago	eat, swallow	phage	_____
		phagocyte	_____
plasia	development or formation	aplasia	_____
		hyperplasia	_____
plasm	the constituent substance of cells	plasmatic	_____
		plasmocytoma	_____
plegia	paralysis; losing feeling in or control of	bronchoplegia	_____
		hemi/semiplegia	_____

-ptosis	drooping	gastroptosis	_____
		nephroptosis	_____
quadri-	four	quadriplegia	_____
		quadrisection	_____
sept-	seven	septet	_____
		septuagenarian	_____
top (o)	part	topalgia	_____
		isotopology	_____
tri-	three	trioxide	_____
		triad	_____
thromb (o)	blood clot	thromboarteritis	_____
		thrombogenesis	_____
troph (o)	nutrition	trophodynamics	_____
		trophotherapy	_____

2. Write down the questions you would like to ask or discuss about the text.

_____

_____

_____

Task Two　Vocabulary

Choose the word or phrase that can best complete the statements.

1) All clinical details, investigation results, discussion of treatment options, informed _____, and treatment by herbal medicines or TCM procedures and prescriptions should be documented.

A. approvals　　　　B. agreements　　　　C. consents　　　　D. complaints

2) A TCM practitioner who _____ his patient of any supporting medical service is responsible for the adequate provision of such supporting medical service and must be reasonably confident of the standard and reliability of that service.

A. ensures　　　　B. avails　　　　C. refers　　　　D. compels

3) There is an unfortunate abundance of intellectual _____ in the broad field of "alternative medicine", a field to which TCM, as practiced in the West, often attaches itself.

A. clarification　　　B. dishonesty　　　C. adaptation　　　D. complexion

4) Patients' health and well-being, as well as their wallets, are affected by weak ethical standards, and the entire profession can be _____ by failing to adhere to high standards.

A. promoted　　　　B. dedicated　　　　C. adjusted　　　　D. tainted

5) Using traditional medicine systems does not require that each _____ of the system be proven valid or effective, because traditional medicine is a cultural construct that is being retained.

A. composition　　　B. ingredient　　　C. component　　　D. participation

6) Well-educated practitioners are more likely to keep to the scope of practice for which they are _____ .

笔记

A. given   B. recognized   C. licensed   D. satisfied

7) A TCM practitioner _____ responsibility for the overall management of the patient when he delegates another TCM practitioner to provide treatment or care on his behalf.

    A. retains   B. restricts   C. pertains   D. manipulates

8) In their enthusiasm for offering these new non-authentic techniques, practitioners may not realize that they are providing a certain _____.

    A. representation   B. deception   C. exclamation   D. implication

9) The field of TCM is still in its infancy in the West, leaving it _____ to negative impressions. Not all states in the country have provision for licensing practitioners.

    A. contagious   B. infectious   C. sensible   D. vulnerable

10) A TCM physician should prescribe, _____ or supply medicines on clear medical grounds and in reasonable quantities as appropriate to the patient's needs.

    A. dispose   B. dispense   C. decompose   D. disrepute

11) It is required that all the practitioners, as the commitment to the patient, protect the _____ of information acquired in the course of medical care.

    A. confidentiality   B. respectability

    C. authoritativeness   D. compatibility

12) Obesity carries an increased risk of _____.

    A. mortality   B. mobility   C. longevity   D. maternity

13) Despite his doctor's note of caution, he never _____ from drinking and smoking.

    A. retained   B. dissuaded   C. alleviated   D. abstained

14) Heat stroke is a medical emergency that demands immediate _____ from qualified medical personnel.

    A. prescription   B. palpation   C. interaction   D. interposition

15) Most colds are acquired by children in school and then _____ to adults.

    A. conveyed   B. transmitted   C. attributed   D. relayed

Task Three   Translation

Translate the following expressions into English.

1) 医学伦理   2) 中医执业者

3) 东方医学   4) 医疗实践

5) 全社会   6) 医疗信息

7) 道德准则   8) 知情同意

9) 道德冲突   10) 参与决定治疗方案

11) 道德修养   12) 知情权

13) 坚守职业精神   14) 隐私权和尊严

15) 公共卫生教育   16) 在严格保密框架下

17) 医学伦理委员会   18) 死亡率

19) 遭受患者亲属任何形式的诋毁   20) 存活率

PART Ⅲ　TRANSLATION AND WRITING

How to Write Ethical Guidelines for Traditional
Chinese Medicine Practitioners

Apart from the laws governing the society, traditional Chinese medicine (TCM) practitioners are obliged to adhere to the ethical guidelines regulating the practice and conduct of the persons registered in the profession. Such professional guidelines usually cover such items as standard of good TCM practice(良好的中医医疗作业标准), relationships with patients(与患者的关系), relationships with fellow TCM practitioners(中医师与同行之间的关系), information about TCM practitioner's services(关于中医师的医疗服务信息), TCM practitioners in non-medical context(在非医疗环境中的中医师), and so on.

TCM practitioner's guidelines should be in written language, and imperatives, sentences with passive voice and modal verbs are usually used. The following sentences or expressions are commonly seen.

1) "The Ethical Guidelines for TCM Practitioners" represents the fundamental tenets of conduct and behavior expected of TCM practitioners practicing in the country and elaborates on their applications.

《中医师道德指导原则》体现了对本国注册中医师操守和行为的基本要求,并且详述了它们的应用。

2) Serious disregard or persistent failure to meet these standards can potentially lead to harm to patients or bring disrepute to the profession and consequently may lead to disciplinary proceedings.

蔑视这些要求或持续不能达到这些要求将可能伤害到患者或破坏中医行业的信誉,结果可能导致纪律诉讼。

3) They are intended as a guide to all TCM practitioners as to what is regarded by the professional board as the minimum standards required of all TCM practitioners in the discharge of their professional duties and responsibilities in the practice of TCM in the country.

目的是让所有中医师了解专业委员会对国内中医师的专业水准和专业责任的最低要求。

4) TCM practitioners are exhorted to keep both the principles and the spirit of this "Ethical Guidelines for TCM Practitioners" firmly in mind in the course of their practice.

中医师在进行医疗工作时,应将此《中医师道德指导原则》的准则和精神牢记在心。

5) A TCM practitioner is expected to have a sense of responsibility for his patients and to provide medical care only after an adequate assessment of a patient's condition through good history taking and appropriate TCM clinical examination.

中医师应该对患者有责任感,在详细了解病史、依据适当的中医临床检查对患者

笔记

203

的病情做出正确诊断后,再进行治疗。

6) A TCM practitioner may delegate another TCM practitioner to provide treatment or care on his behalf, but this person must be competent to carry out the care or procedure required and the patient's well-being, treatment and safety are not compromised. In any event, the TCM practitioner is ultimately answerable for the treatment or care provided to such patient(s).

中医师可以委托另一位中医师为患者提供治疗或照顾,但接受委托之人必须有能力胜任所委托的职责,不危害患者的健康、治疗和安全。在任何情况下,该中医师必须对为患者提供的治疗和照顾负责。

7) A TCM practitioner should practice within the limits of his own competence in managing a patient. A TCM practitioner shall not persist in unsupervised practice of a branch of medicine without having the appropriate knowledge and skill or having the required experience.

中医师应在其能力范围内为患者诊治。若在某个方面缺乏应有的知识、技能或所需的经验,中医师不应该在没有监督的情况下坚持为患者进行治疗。

8) A TCM practitioner shall ensure that proper and accurate records are kept to enable proper aftercare and service for his patients, and the medical records shall include the particulars of the patients and shall be clear, accurate, and legible and shall be made at the time that a consultation takes place.

中医师应该保存完整和准确的病历,以便为患者提供复诊服务。所保存的病历应包括患者的个人详情,记录必须书写清楚、准确,字体容易辨读。病历应是在诊治时记录。

9) A TCM physician may only prescribe herbal medicines that are legally available in the country and must comply with all relevant statutory requirements governing their use.

中医师只能使用在本国可以合法使用的中草药来开方配药,并且必须遵守管制药物使用的法令。

10) Patients shall be appropriately informed about the purpose of the prescribed medicines, method of preparation, dosage, contraindications and possible side effects.

中医师应向患者适当说明所开配药物的用途、煎煮方法、剂量、禁忌和可能产生的副作用。

11) It is a TCM practitioner's responsibility to ensure that a patient under his care is adequately informed about his medical condition and options for treatment so that he is able to participate in decisions about his treatment.

中医师有责任确保患者在接受治疗的过程中,能够了解自身病况和可供选择的治疗方案,使患者能够参与决定治疗方法。

12) A TCM practitioner shall respect the principle of medical confidentiality and not disclose without a patient's consent, information obtained in confidence or in the course of attending to the patient.

中医师应该尊重医疗保密的原则。私下或在医治患者时获得的患者个人资料,未经患者同意不得泄露。

13) A TCM practitioner shall refrain from making gratuitous and unsustainable comments which, whether expressly or by implication, set out to undermine the trust in a professional colleague's knowledge or skills in TCM.

中医师应避免以直接或影射的方式对同业者做出无来由的、没有根据的评论，以免破坏人们对该同业者的专业知识或技能的信任。

14) TCM practitioners can validly provide information about the services they provide to both colleagues and members of the public. However, such provision of information shall not become blatant advertising in the commercial sense of the word as this could mislead patients, undermine trust and be demeaning to the profession.

中医师可以正当地提供服务信息给其同业者和公众。不过，这些信息不得含有商业性广告的意味，因为这会误导患者，破坏患者对中医师的信任并降低中医行业的形象。

15) A TCM practitioner shall not carry on trade, business or calling that is incompatible with or detracts from the practice of TCM and brings his practice and his profession into disrepute.

中医师不应从事与专业不相容，或会令其对专业分心和有损其专业声誉的贸易、商业或集会活动。

Sample

Chinese Doctor Code of Ethics

Chinese Doctor Code of Ethics, formulated and issued by Chinese Medical Doctor Association in June 2014, stipulates the basic moral code that Chinese doctors should abide by. 1) The code of ethics is intended to regulate the moral bottom line of doctors, promote doctors to sublimate their professional means of livelihood into professional faith, and require doctors to comply with the requirements of professional self-discipline and win the respect of the society.

In terms of the relationship between doctors and patients, the code of ethics requires that doctors should treat patients with full respect and give them proper care with compassion. Doctors are expected to communicate with the patient in language or manner that the patient can understand, and answer the questions raised by the patient as much as possible, not to mislead or attract patients by false propaganda or improper means, and not to harm patients or put patients in unnecessary risk situations with medical knowledge and professional technology. 2) Informed consent before surgery, special examination and treatment should not be regarded as a waiver or self-protection initiative, and should not be regarded as a mere formality or burden. In terms of doctors and enterprises, 3) the code of ethics stipulates that doctors should not conduct scientific and ethical research on the basis of financial support from pharmaceutical enterprises, nor promote any medical products or academic promotion for personal benefit.

As is specified in the code of ethics, doctors should deal well with the relationship with patients, colleagues, society and enterprises, and 4) they are encouraged to pursue

笔记

lifelong learning, to improve constantly their expertise and skills, and to allocate medical resources in a fair and equitable manner to maximize their benefits. 5) They should carry forward the humanistic spirit and strengthen professional ethics, and should be committed to responsible and ethical practice, to their own professional growth, as well as the development of China's health care.

Task One　Translation

Translate the underlined parts in the above sample into Chinese.

1) _____

_____

_____

2) _____

_____

_____

3) _____

_____

_____

4) _____

_____

_____

5) _____

_____

_____

Task Two　Writing

Write 10-15 ethical rules or guidelines for TCM practitioners based on your understanding of this profession. Try to use as many sentence patterns as possible in PART Ⅲ. Alternatively, you may work in pairs on this issue, search the information on the internet, write the guidelines and then present them to the class.

_____

_____

_____

PART IV   REFLECTION

You are a general medical practitioner in the United Sates. A mother comes into your office with her child who is complaining of flu-like symptoms. You ask the boy to remove his shirt for examination and you notice a pattern of very distinct bruises on the boy's torso. The mother tells you that they are from a procedure she performed on him known as *"guasha"*. The procedure involves rubbing warm oils or gels on a person's skin with a coin or other flat metal object. According to the mother, *guasha* is often used in TCM to remove bad blood, and improve circulation and healing. When you touch the boy's back with your stethoscope, he winces in pain from the bruises. Please debate whether or not you should call Child Protective Services and accuse the mother of abusing the child.

Questions for you to think about:

1) Should you completely discount *guasha* as useless, or could there be something that you can learn from it?

2) When should you (a physician) step in to stop a cultural practice?

Appendix I

Traditional Chinese Medicine Book Titles

序号	古籍名称	世中联版本 [1]	WHO 版本 [2]	名词委版本 [3]
1	《备急千金要方》	*Important Prescriptions Worth a Thousand Gold for Emergency*	*Essential Prescriptions Worth a Thousand Gold for Emergencies*	*Beiji Qianjin Yao Fang; Essential Recipes for Emergent Use Worth A Thousand Gold*
2	《本草纲目》	*Compendium of Materia Medica*	*Compendium of Materia Medica*	*Bencao Gangmu; Compendium of Materia Medica*
3	《本草纲目拾遗》	*Supplement to Compendium of Materia Medica*	*Supplement to the Compendium of Materia Medica*	*Bencao Gangmu Shiyi; Supplement to Compendium of Materia Medica*
4	《濒湖脉学》	*Binhu's Sphygmology*	*Binhu's Sphygmology*	—
5	《丹溪心法》	*Danxi's Experiential Therapy*	*Danxi's Experiential Therapy*	*Danxi Xinfa; Danxi's Mastery of Medicine*
6	《妇人大全良方》	*A Complete Collection of Effective Prescriptions for Women*	*Compendium of Effective Prescriptions for Women*	*Furen Daquan Liang Fang; Complete Effective Prescriptions for Women's Diseases*
7	《格致余论》	*Further Discourses on Acquiring Knowledge by Studying Properties of Things*	*Treatise on Inquiring the Properties of Things*	*Gezhi Yu Lun; Further Discourses on the Properties of Things*

续表

序号	古籍名称	世中联版本 [1]	WHO 版本 [2]	名词委版本 [3]
8	《古今医统大全》	Medical Complete Books, Ancient and Modern	Complete Compendium of Medical Works, Ancient and Modern	Gujin Yitong Daquan; Medical Complete Book, Ancient and Modern
9	《黄帝内经》	Huangdi's Internal Classic	Huangdi's Internal Classic	Huangdi Neijing; Inner Canon of Huangdi; Inner Canon of Yellow Emperor
10	《济阴纲目》	Outline for Women's Diseases	Synopsis of Treating Women's Diseases	Ji Yin Gangmu; Outline for Women's Diseases
11	《金匮要略》	Synopsis of the Golden Chamber	Synopsis of Prescriptions of the Golden Chamber	Jingui Yaolüe; Synopsis of Golden Chamber
12	《经史证类备急本草》	Classified Materia Medica from Historical Classics for Emergency	Classified Emergency Materia Medica	Jing Shi Zheng Lei Beiji Bencao; Classified Materia Medica from Historical Classics for Emergency
13	《救荒本草》	Materia Medica for Famine Relief	Materia Medica for Relief of Famines	Jiuhuang Bencao; Materia Medica for Famines
14	《局方发挥》	Expounding of Prescriptions of the Bureau of Pharmacy	Elucidation of Dispensary Formulas	Jufang Fahui; Elaboration of Bureau Prescription
15	《兰室秘藏》	Secret Book of the Orchid Chamber	Secret Records of the Orchid Chamber	Lanshi Micang; Secret Book of Orchid Chamber
16	《雷公炮炙论》	Master Lei's Discourse on Medicinal Processing	Lei's Treatise on Processing of Drugs	Leigong Paozhi Lun; Master Lei's Discourse on Drug Processing
17	《类经》	Classified Classic	Classified Classic	Lei Jing; Classified Canon
18	《刘涓子鬼遗方》	Liu Juanzi's Ghost-Bequeathed Prescriptions	Liu Juanzi's Ghost-Bequeathed Prescriptions	Liu Juanzi Guiyi Fang; Liu Juanzi's Remedies Bequeathed by Ghosts

续表

序号	古籍名称	世中联版本 [1]	WHO 版本 [2]	名词委版本 [3]
19	《脉经》	Pulse Classic	Pulse Classic	Mai Jing; Pulse Classic
20	《秘传眼科龙木论》	Longmu's Ophthalmology Secretly Handed Down	Nagarjuna's Secret Treatise on Ophthalmology	Michuan Yanke Longmu Lun; Nagarjuna's Ophthalmology Secretly Handed Down
21	《难经》	Classic of Difficulties	Classic of Difficult Issues	Nan Jing; Classic of Questioning
22	《脾胃论》	Treatise on Spleen and Stomach	Treatise on the Spleen and Stomach	Piwei Lun; Treatise on Spleen and Stomach
23	《普济本事方》	Experiential Prescriptions for Universal Relief	Moxibustion in Prescriptions for Universal Relief	—
24	《千金翼方》	Supplement to Prescriptions Worth a Thousand Gold Pieces	Supplement to the Essential Prescriptions Worth a Thousand Gold	Qianjin Yi Fang; A Supplement to Recipes Worth A Thousand Gold
25	《儒门事亲》	Confucians' Duties to Parents	Confucians' Duties to Their Parents	Rumen Shi Qin; Confucians' Duties to Parents
26	《三因极 - 病证方论》	Treatise on Diseases, Patterns, and Prescriptions Related to Unification of the Three Etiologies	Treatise on the Three Categories of Pathogenic Factors and Prescriptions	—
27	《伤寒论》	Treatise on Cold Damage	Treatise on Cold Damage Diseases	Shanghan Lun; Treatise on Cold Pathogenic Diseases
28	《伤寒杂病论》	Treatise on Cold Damage and Miscellaneous Diseases	Treatise on Cold Damage and Miscellaneous Diseases	Shanghan Zabing Lun; Treatise on Cold Pathogenic and Miscellaneous Diseases
29	《神农本草经》	Shennong's Classic of Materia Medica	Shennong's Classic of Materia Medica	Shennong Bencao Jing; Shennong's Classic of Materia Medica

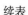

续表

序号	古籍名称	世中联版本 [1]	WHO 版本 [2]	名词委版本 [3]
30	《审视瑶函》	Precious Book of Ophthalmology	Compendium of Ophthalmology	Shen Shi Yao Han; Precious Book of Ophthalmology
31	《圣济总录 》	Comprehensive Recording of Sage-like Benefit	Complete Record of Sacred Benevolence	Sheng Ji Zonglu; General Records of Holy Universe Relief
32	《时病论》	Discussion of Seasonal Diseases	Treatise on Seasonal Epidemic Diseases	—
33	《食疗本草》	Materia Medica for Dietotherapy	Dietetic Materia Medica	Shiliao Bencao; Materia Medica for Dietotherapy
34	《太平惠民和剂局方》	Formulary of the Bureau of Taiping People's Welfare Pharmacy	Prescriptions from the Great Peace Imperial Grace Pharmacy	Taiping Huimin Heji Ju Fang; Prescriptions of the Bureau of Taiping People's Welfare Pharmacy
35	《太平圣惠方》	Taiping Holy Prescriptions for Universal Relief	Peaceful Holy Benevolent Prescriptions	Taiping Shenghui Fang; Taiping Holy Prescriptions for Universal Relief
36	《汤头歌诀》	Prescriptions in Rhymes	Prescriptions in Rhymes	Tangtou Gejue; Recipes in Rhymes
37	《铜人俞穴针灸图经》	Illustrated Manual of Acupoints of the Bronze Figure	Illustrated Manual of Acupuncture Points of the Bronze Figure	—
38	《外科精要》	Essence of External Diseases	Essentials of External Medicine	Waike Jingyao; Essence of External Diseases
39	《外科正宗》	Orthodox Manual of External Medicine	Orthodox Manual of External Medicine	Waike Zhengzong; Orthodox Manual of External Diseases
40	《温病条辨》	Detailed Analysis of Warm Diseases	Systematized Identification of Warm (Pathogen) Diseases	Wenbing Tiaobian; Detailed Analysis of Epidemic Warm Diseases
41	《温热经纬》	Warp and Woof of Warm-Heat Diseases	Warp and Weft of Warm Heat Disease	—

续表

序号	古籍名称	世中联版本 [1]	WHO 版本 [2]	名词委版本 [3]
42	《温热论》	Treatise on Warm-Heat Diseases	Treatise on Warm Heat Disease	—
43	《温疫论》	Treatise on Pestilence	Treatise on Pestilence	Wenyi Lun; On Plague Disease
44	《小儿药证直诀》	Key to Medicines and Patterns of Children's Diseases	Key to Therapeutics of Children's Diseases	Xiao'er Yao Zheng Zhi Jue; Key to Therapeutics of Children's Diseases
45	《新修本草》	Newly Revised Materia Medica	Newly Revised Materia Medica (Tang Materia Medica)	Xinxiu Bencao; Newly Revised Materia Medica
46	《血证论》	Treatise on Blood Syndromes	Treatise on Blood Patterns/Syndromes	Xuezheng Lun; On Blood Syndromes
47	《医贯》	Key Link of Medicine	Thorough Knowledge of Medicine	Yi Guan; Key Link of Medicine
48	《医林改错》	Correction on Errors in Medical Works	Correction of Errors in Medical Classics	Yilin Gaicuo; Correction of Errors in Medical Classics
49	《医门法律》	Precepts for Physicians	Principles for Medical Profession	—
50	《医学入门》	Introduction to Medicine	Introduction to Medicine	
51	《医学心悟》	Comprehension of Medicine	Medical Insights	
52	《医学正传》	Orthodox Lineage of Medicine（《医学正宗》）	Orthodox Transmission of Medicine	—
53	《医宗必读》	Required Readings from the Medical Ancestors	Required Readings for Medical Professionals	—
54	《医宗金鉴》	Golden Mirror of the Medical Ancestors	Golden Mirror of Medicine	Yizong Jinjian; Golden Mirror of Medicine
55	《银海精微》	Essentials of Ophthalmology	Essence on the Silvery Sea	—
56	《幼幼集成》	Complete Work on Children's Diseases	Compendium of Pediatrics	Youyou Jicheng; Complete Work on Children's Diseases

续表

序号	古籍名称	世中联版本 [1]	WHO 版本 [2]	名词委版本 [3]
57	《幼幼新书》	New Book of Pediatrics	New Book of Pediatrics	Youyou Xin Shu; New Book of Pediatrics
58	《针灸大成》	Great Compendium of Acupuncture and Moxibustion	Complete Compendium of Acupuncture and Moxibustion	Zhenjiu Dacheng; Compendium of Acupuncture and Moxibustion
59	《针灸甲乙经》	A-B Classic of Acupuncture and Moxibustion	A-B Classic of Acupuncture and Moxibustion	Zhenjiu Jiayi Jing; A-B Classic of Acupuncture and Moxibustion
60	《针灸聚英》	A Collection of Gems in Acupuncture and Moxibustion	Collection of Gems of Acupuncture and Moxibustion	—
61	《针灸资生经》	Classic of Nourishing Life with Acupuncture and Moxibustion	Classic of Nourishing Life with Acupuncture and Moxibustion	—
62	《证治准绳》	Criterion for Pattern Identification and Treatment	Standards of Pattern/Syndrome Identification and Treatment	Zhengzhi Zhunsheng; Standards for Diagnosis and Treatment
63	《肘后备急方》	Handbook of Prescriptions for Emergency	Handbook of Prescriptions for Emergencies	Zhouhou Beiji Fang; Handbook of Prescriptions for Emergency
64	《诸病源候论》	Treatise on Causes and Manifestations of Various Diseases	Treatise on the Pathogenesis and Manifestations of All Diseases	Zhu Bing Yuan Hou Lun; General Treatise on Causes and Manifestation of All Diseases

参考书目

[1] 李振吉. 中医基本名词术语中英对照国际标准 [M]. 北京：人民卫生出版社，2008

[2] WHO Western Pacific Region. WHO international standard terminologies on traditional Chinese medicine in the Western Pacific region[M]. Geneva: World Health Organization, 2007

[3] 全国科学技术名词审定委员会. 中医药学名词 (2004) [M]. 北京：科学出版社，2005

Appendix II

Acupoints

手太阴肺经穴 Shǒutàiyīn Fèijīng Xué
Points of Lung Meridian of Hand-Taiyin, LU

中府[Zhōngfǔ]（LU1）
云门[Yúnmén]（LU2）
天府[Tiānfǔ]（LU3）
侠白[Xiábái]（LU4）
尺泽[Chǐzé]（LU5）
孔最[Kǒngzuì]（LU6）
列缺[Lièquē]（LU7）
经渠[Jīngqú]（LU8）
太渊[Tàiyuān]（LU9）
鱼际[Yújì]（LU10）
少商[Shàoshāng]（LU11）

手阳明大肠经穴 Shǒuyángmíng Dàchángjīng Xué
Points of Large Intestine Meridian of Hand-Yangming, LI

商阳[Shāngyáng]（LI1）
二间[èrjiān]（LI2）
三间[Sānjiān]（LI3）
合谷[Hégǔ]（LI4）
阳溪[Yángxī]（LI5）
偏历[Piānlì]（LI6）
温溜[Wēnliū]（LI7）
下廉[Xiàlián]（LI8）
上廉[Shànglián]（LI9）
手三里[Shǒusānlǐ]（LI10）
曲池[Qūchí]（LI11）

肘髎[Zhǒuliáo]（LI12）
手五里[Shǒuwǔlǐ]（LI13）
臂臑[Bìnào]（LI14）
肩髃[Jiānyú]（LI15）
巨骨[Jùgǔ]（LI16）
天鼎[Tiāndǐng]（LI17）
扶突[Fútū]（LI18）
口禾髎[Kǒuhéliáo]（LI19）
迎香[Yíngxiāng]（LI20）

足阳明胃经穴 Zúyángmíng Wèijīng Xué
Points of Stomach Meridian of Foot-Yangming, ST

承泣[Chéngqì]（ST1）
四白[Sìbái]（ST2）
巨髎[Jùliáo]（ST3）
地仓[Dìcāng]（ST4）
大迎[Dàyíng]（ST5）
颊车[Jiáchē]（ST6）
下关[Xiàguān]（ST7）
头维[Tóuwéi]（ST8）
人迎[Rényíng]（ST9）
水突[Shuǐtū]（ST10）
气舍[Qìshè]（ST11）
缺盆[Quēpén]（ST12）
气户[Qìhù]（ST13）
库房[Kùfáng]（ST14）
屋翳[Wūyì]（ST15）
膺窗[Yīngchuāng]（ST16）
乳中[Rǔzhōng]（ST17）
乳根[Rǔgēn]（ST18）

不容[Bùróng]（ST19）

承满[Chéngmǎn]（ST20）

梁门[Liángmén]（ST21）

关门[Guānmén]（ST22）

太乙[Tàiyǐ]（ST23）

滑肉门[Huáròumén]（ST24）

天枢[Tiānshū]（ST25）

外陵[Wàilíng]（ST26）

大巨[Dàjù]（ST27）

水道[Shuǐdào]（ST28）

归来[Guīlái]（ST29）

气冲[Qìchōng]（ST30）

髀关[Bìguān]（ST31）

伏兔[Fútù]（ST32）

阴市[Yīnshì]（ST33）

梁丘[Liángqiū]（ST34）

犊鼻[Dúbí]（ST35）

足三里[Zúsānlǐ]（ST36）

上巨虚[Shàngjùxū]（ST37）

条口[Tiáokǒu]（ST38）

下巨虚[Xiàjùxū]（ST39）

丰隆[Fēnglóng]（ST40）

解溪[Jiěxī]（ST41）

冲阳[Chōngyáng]（ST42）

陷谷[Xiàngǔ]（ST43）

内庭[Nèitíng]（ST44）

厉兑[Lìduì]（ST45）

足太阴脾经穴 Zútàiyīn Píjīng Xué Points of Spleen Meridian of Foot-Taiyin, SP

隐白[Yǐnbái]（SP1）

大都[Dàdū]（SP2）

太白[Tàibái]（SP3）

公孙[Gōngsūn]（SP4）

商丘[Shāngqiū]（SP5）

三阴交[Sānyīnjiāo]（SP6）

漏谷[Lòugǔ]（SP7）

地机[Dìjī]（SP8）

阴陵泉[Yīnlíngquán]（SP9）

血海[Xuèhǎi]（SP10）

箕门[Jīmén]（SP11）

冲门[Chōngmén]（SP12）

府舍[Fǔshè]（SP13）

腹结[Fùjié]（SP14）

大横[Dàhéng]（SP15）

腹哀[Fù'āi]（SP16）

食窦[Shídòu]（SP17）

天溪[Tiānxī]（SP18）

胸乡[Xiōngxiāng]（SP19）

周荣[Zhōuróng]（SP20）

大包[Dàbāo]（SP21）

手少阴心经穴 Shǒushàoyīn Xīnjīng Xué Points of Heart Meridian of Hand-Shaoyin, HT

极泉[Jíquán]（HT1）

青灵[Qīnglíng]（HT2）

少海[Shàohǎi]（HT3）

灵道[Língdào]（HT4）

通里[Tōnglǐ]（HT5）

阴郄[Yīnxì]（HT6）

神门[Shénmén]（HT7）

少府[Shàofǔ]（HT8）

少冲[Shàochōng]（HT9）

手太阳小肠经穴 Shǒutàiyáng Xiǎochángjīng Xué Points of Small Intestine Meridian of Hand-Taiyang, SI

少泽[Shàozé]（SI1）

前谷[Qiángǔ]（SI2）

后溪[Hòuxī]（SI3）

腕骨[Wàngǔ]（SI4）

阳谷[Yánggǔ]（SI5）

养老[Yǎnglǎo]（SI6）

支正[Zhīzhèng]（SI7）

小海[Xiǎohǎi]（SI8）

肩贞[Jiānzhēn]（SI9）

臑俞[Nàoshū]（SI10）

天宗[Tiānzōng]（SI11）

秉风[Bǐngfēng]（SI12）

曲垣[Qūyuán]（SI13）

肩外俞[Jiānwàishū]（SI14）

肩中俞[Jiānzhōngshū]（SI15）

天窗[Tiānchuāng]（SI16）

天容［Tiānróng］（SI17）
颧髎［Quánliáo］（SI18）
听宫［Tīnggōng］（SI19）

足太阳膀胱经穴 Zútàiyáng Pángguāngjīng Xué
Points of Bladder Meridian of Foot-Taiyang, BL

睛明［Jīngmíng］（BL1）
攒竹［Cuánzhú］（BL2）
眉冲［Méichōng］（BL3）
曲差［Qūchā］（BL4）
五处［Wǔchù］（BL5）
承光［Chéngguāng］（BL6）
通天［Tōngtiān］（BL7）
络却［Luòquè］（BL8）
玉枕［Yùzhěn］（BL9）
天柱［Tiānzhù］（BL10）
大杼［Dàzhù］（BL11）
风门［Fēngmén］（BL12）
肺俞［Fèishū］（BL13）
厥阴俞［Juéyīnshū］（BL14）
心俞［Xīnshū］（BL15）
督俞［Dūshū］（BL16）
膈俞［Géshū］（BL17）
肝俞［Gānshū］（BL18）
胆俞［Dǎnshū］（BL19）
脾俞［Píshū］（BL20）
胃俞［Wèishū］（BL21）
三焦俞［Sānjiāoshū］（BL22）
肾俞［Shènshū］（BL23）
气海俞［Qìhǎishū］（BL24）
大肠俞［Dàchángshū］（BL25）
关元俞［Guānyuánshū］（BL26）
小肠俞［Xiǎochángshū］（BL27）
膀胱俞［Pángguāngshū］（BL28）
中膂俞［Zhōnglǚshū］（BL29）
白环俞［Báihuánshū］（BL30）
上髎［Shàngliáo］（BL31）
次髎［Cìliáo］（BL32）
中髎［Zhōngliáo］（BL33）
下髎［Xiàliáo］（BL34）
会阳［Huìyáng］（BL35）

承扶［Chéngfú］（BL36）
殷门［Yīnmén］（BL37）
浮郄［Fúxì］（BL38）
委阳［Wěiyáng］（BL39）
委中［Wěizhōng］（BL40）
附分［Fùfēn］（BL41）
魄户［Pòhù］（BL42）
膏肓［Gāohuāng］（BL43）
神堂［Shéntáng］（BL44）
谚语［Yìxǐ］（BL45）
膈关［Géguān］（BL46）
魂门［Húnmén］（BL47）
阳纲［Yánggāng］（BL48）
意舍［Yìshè］（BL49）
胃仓［Wèicāng］（BL50）
肓门［Huāngmén］（BL51）
志室［Zhìshì］（BL52）
胞肓［Bāohuāng］（BL53）
秩边［Zhìbiān］（BL54）
合阳［Héyáng］（BL55）
承筋［Chéngjīn］（BL56）
承山［Chéngshān］（BL57）
飞扬［Fēiyáng］（BL58）
跗阳［Fūyáng］（BL59）
昆仑［Kūnlún］（BL60）
仆参［Púcān］（BL61）
申脉［Shēnmài］（BL62）
金门［Jīnmén］（BL63）
京骨［Jīnggǔ］（BL64）
束骨［Shùgǔ］（BL65）
足通谷［Zútōnggǔ］（BL66）
至阴［Zhìyīn］（BL67）

足少阴肾经穴 Zúshàoyīn Shènjīng Xué
Points of Kidney Meridian of Foot-Shaoyin, KI

涌泉［Yǒngquán］（KI1）
然谷［Rángǔ］（KI2）
太溪［Tàixī］（KI3）
大钟［Dàzhōng］（KI4）
水泉［Shuǐquán］（KI5）
照海［Zhàohǎi］（KI6）
复溜［Fùliū］（KI7）

交信[Jiāoxìn]（KI8）

筑宾[Zhùbīn]（KI9）

阴谷[Yīngǔ]（KI10）

横骨[Hénggǔ]（KI11）

大赫[Dàhè]（KI12）

气穴[Qìxué]（KI13）

四满[Sìmǎn]（KI14）

中注[Zhōngzhù]（KI15）

肓俞[Huāngshū]（KI16）

商曲[Shāngqū]（KI17）

石关[Shíguān]（KI18）

阴都[Yīndū]（KI19）

腹通谷[Fùtōnggǔ]（KI20）

幽门[Yōumén]（KI21）

步廊[Bùláng]（KI22）

神封[Shénfēng]（KI23）

灵墟[Língxū]（KI24）

神藏[Shéncáng]（KI25）

彧中[Yùzhōng]（KI26）

俞府[Shūfǔ]（KI27）

手厥阴心包经穴 Shǒujuéyīn Xīnbāojīng Xué Points of Pericardium Meridian of Hand-Jueyin, PC

天池[Tiānchí]（PC1）

天泉[Tiānquán]（PC2）

曲泽[Qūzé]（PC3）

郄门[Xìmén]（PC4）

间使[Jiānshǐ]（PC5）

内关[Nèiguān]（PC6）

大陵[Dàlíng]（PC7）

劳宫[Láogōng]（PC8）

中冲[Zhōngchōng]（PC9）

手少阳三焦经穴 Shǒushàoyáng Sānjiāojīng Xué Points of Triple Energizer Meridian of Hand-Shaoyang, TE

关冲[Guānchōng]（TE1）

液门[Yèmén]（TE2）

中渚[Zhōngzhǔ]（TE3）

阳池[Yángchí]（TE4）

外关[Wàiguān]（TE5）

支沟[Zhīgōu]（TE6）

会宗[Huìzōng]（TE7）

三阳络[Sānyángluò]（TE8）

四渎[Sìdú]（TE9）

天井[Tiānjǐng]（TE10）

清冷渊[Qīnglěngyuān]（TE11）

消泺[Xiāoluò]（TE12）

臑会[Nàohuì]（TE13）

肩髎[Jiānliáo]（TE14）

天髎[Tiānliáo]（TE15）

天牖[Tiānyǒu]（TE16）

翳风[Yìfēng]（TE17）

瘈脉[Chìmài]（TE18）

颅息[Lúxī]（TE19）

角孙[Jiǎosūn]（TE20）

耳门[ěrmén]（TE21）

耳和髎[ěrhéliáo]（TE22）

丝竹空[Sīzhúkōng]（TE23）

足少阳胆经穴 Zúshàoyáng Dǎnjīng Xué Points of Gallbladder Meridian of Foot-Shaoyang, GB

瞳子髎[Tóngzǐliáo]（GB1）

听会[Tīnghuì]（GB2）

上关[Shàngguān]（GB3）

颔厌[Hànyàn]（GB4）

悬颅[Xuánlú]（GB5）

悬厘[Xuánlí]（GB6）

曲鬓[Qūbìn]（GB7）

率谷[Shuàigǔ]（GB8）

天冲[Tiānchōng]（GB9）

浮白[Fúbái]（GB10）

头窍阴[Tóuqiàoyīn]（GB11）

完骨[Wángǔ]（GB12）

本神[Běnshén]（GB13）

阳白[Yángbái]（GB14）

头临泣[Tóulínqì]（GB15）

目窗[Mùchuāng]（GB16）

正营[Zhèngyíng]（GB17）

承灵[Chénglíng]（GB18）

脑空[Nǎokōng]（GB19）

风池[Fēngchí]（GB20）

肩井[Jiānjǐng]（GB21）

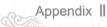

渊腋［Yuānyè］（GB22）
辄筋［Zhéjīn］（GB23）
日月［Rìyuè］（GB24）
京门［Jīngmén］（GB25）
带脉［Dàimài］（GB26）
五枢［Wǔshū］（GB27）
维道［Wéidào］（GB28）
居髎［Jūliáo］（GB29）
环跳［Huántiào］（GB30）
风市［Fēngshì］（GB31）
中渎［Zhōngdú］（GB32）
膝阳关［Xīyángguān］（GB33）
阳陵泉［Yánglíngquán］（GB34）
阳交［Yángjiāo］（GB35）
外丘［Wàiqiū］（GB36）
光明［Guāngmíng］（GB37）
阳辅［Yángfǔ］（GB38）
悬钟［Xuánzhōng］（GB39）
丘墟［Qiūxū］（GB40）
足临泣［Zúlínqì］（GB41）
地五会［Dìwǔhuì］（GB42）
侠溪［Xiáxī］（GB43）
足窍阴［Zúqiàoyīn］（GB44）

足厥阴肝经穴 Zújuéyīn Gānjīng Xué
Points of Liver Meridian of Foot-Jueyin, LR

大敦［Dàdūn］（LR1）
行间［Xíngjiān］（LR2）
太冲［Tàichōng］（LR3）
中封［Zhōngfēng］（LR4）
蠡沟［Lígōu］（LR5）
中都［Zhōngdū］（LR6）
膝关［Xīguān］（LR7）
曲泉［Qūquán］（LR8）
阴包［Yīnbāo］（LR9）
足五里［Zúwǔlǐ］（LR10）
阴廉［Yīnlián］（LR11）
急脉［Jímài］（LR12）
章门［Zhāngmén］（LR13）
期门［Qīmén］（LR14）

督脉穴 Dūmài Xué
Points of Governor Vessel, GV

长强［Chángqiáng］（GV1）
腰俞［Yāoshū］（GV2）
腰阳关［Yāoyángguān］（GV3）
命门［Mìngmén］（GV4）
悬枢［Xuánshū］（GV5）
脊中［Jǐzhōng］（GV6）
中枢［Zhōngshū］（GV7）
筋缩［Jīnsuō］（GV8）
至阳［Zhìyáng］（GV9）
灵台［Língtái］（GV10）
神道［Shéndào］（GV11）
身柱［Shēnzhù］（GV12）
陶道［Táodào］（GV13）
大椎［Dàzhuī］（GV14）
哑门［Yǎmén］（GV15）
风府［Fēngfǔ］（GV16）
脑户［Nǎohù］（GV17）
强间［Qiángjiān］（GV18）
后顶［Hòudǐng］（GV19）
百会［Bǎihuì］（GV20）
前顶［Qiándǐng］（GV21）
囟会［Xìnhuì］（GV22）
上星［Shàngxīng］（GV23）
神庭［Shéntíng］（GV24）
素髎［Sùliáo］（GV25）
水沟［Shuǐgōu］（GV26）
兑端［Duìduān］（GV27）
龈交［Yínjiāo］（GV28）

任脉穴 Rénmài Xué
Points of Conception Vessel, CV

会阴［Huìyīn］（CV1）
曲骨［Qūgǔ］（CV2）
中极［Zhōngjí］（CV3）
关元［Guānyuán］（CV4）
石门［Shímén］（CV5）
气海［Qìhǎi］（CV6）
阴交［Yīnjiāo］（CV7）
神阙［Shénquè］（CV8）
水分［Shuǐfēn］（CV9）

下脘［Xiàwǎn］（CV10）
建里［Jiànlǐ］（CV11）
中脘［Zhōngwǎn］（CV12）
上脘［Shàngwǎn］（CV13）
巨阙［Jùquè］（CV14）
鸠尾［Jiūwěi］（CV15）
中庭［Zhōngtíng］（CV16）
膻中［Dànzhōng］（CV17）
玉堂［Yùtáng］（CV18）
紫宫［Zǐgōng］（CV19）
华盖［Huágài］（CV20）
璇玑［Xuánjī］（CV21）
天突［Tiāntū］（CV22）
廉泉［Liánquán］（CV23）
承浆［Chéngjiāng］（CV24）

经外奇穴标准定位 Jīngwài Qíxué Biāozhǔn Dìngwèi
Standard Location of Extra Points, EX

头颈部穴 Tóujǐngbù Xué
Points of Head and Neck, EX-HN
四神聪［Sìshéncōng］（EX-HN1）
当阳［Dāngyáng］（EX-HN2）
印堂［Yìntáng］（EX-HN3）
鱼腰［Yúyāo］（EX-HN4）
太阳［Tàiyáng］（EX-HN5）
耳尖［Ěrjiān］（EX-HN6）
球后［Qiúhòu］（EX-HN7）
上迎香［Shàngyíngxiāng］（EX-HN8）
内迎香［Nèiyíngxiāng］（EX-HN9）
聚泉［Jùquán］（EX-HN10）
海泉［Hǎiquán］（EX-HN11）
金津［Jīnjīn］（EX-HN12）
玉液［Yùyè］（EX-HN13）
翳明［Yìmíng］（EX-HN14）
颈百劳［Jǐngbǎiláo］（EX-HN15）

胸腹部穴 Xiōngfùbù Xué
Points of Chest and Abdomen, EX-CA

子宫［Zǐgōng］（EX-CA1）

背部穴 Bèibù Xué
Points of Back, EX-B

定喘［Dìngchuǎn］（EX-B1）
夹脊［Jiájǐ］（EX-B2）
胃脘下俞［Wèiwǎnxiàshū］（EX-B3）
痞根［Pǐgēn］（EX-B4）
下极俞［Xiàjíshū］（EX-B5）
腰宜［Yāoyí］（EX-B6）
腰眼［Yāoyǎn］（EX-B7）
十七椎［Shíqīzhuī］（EX-B8）
腰奇［Yāoqí］（EX-B9）

上肢穴 Shàngzhī Xué
Points of Upper Extremities, EX-UE

肘尖［Zhǒujiān］（EX-UE1）
二白［Èrbái］（EX-UE2）
中泉［Zhōngquán］（EX-UE3）
中魁［Zhōngkuí］（EX-UE4）
大骨空［Dàgǔkōng］（EX-UE5）
小骨空［Xiǎogǔkōng］（EX-UE6）
腰痛点［Yāotòngdiǎn］（EX-UE7）
外劳宫［Wàiláogōng］（EX-UE8）
八邪［Bāxié］（EX-UE9）
四缝［Sìfèng］（EX-UE10）
十宣［Shíxuān］（EX-UE11）

下肢穴 Xiàzhī Xué
Points of Lower Extremities, EX-LE

髋骨［Kuāngǔ］（EX-LE1）
鹤顶［Hèdǐng］（EX-LE2）
百虫窝［Bǎichóngwō］（EX-LE3）
内膝眼［Nèixīyǎn］（EX-LE4）
膝眼［Xīyǎn］（EX-LE5）
胆囊［Dǎnnáng］（EX-LE6）
阑尾［Lánwěi］（EX-LE7）
内踝尖［Nèihuáijiān］（EX-LE8）
外踝尖［Wèihuáijiān］（EX-LE9）
八风［Bāfēng］（EX-LE10）
独阴［Dúyīn］（EX-LE11）
气端［Qìduān］（EX-LE12）

Appendix Ⅲ

Glossary

Words	POS	Definition and Chinese Meaning	Unit
abdomen /ˈæbdəmən/	*n.*	the part of the body of a vertebrate containing the digestive and reproductive organs; the belly 腹部	2A
abdominal /æbˈdɒmɪn(ə)l/	*a.*	relating to or connected with the abdomen 腹部的	4A
abreast /əˈbrest/	*ad.*	side by side and facing the same way, (usually *abreast of*) alongside or level with sth. 并排地	8B
accordingly /əˈkɔːdɪŋli/	*ad.*	as a result; therefore 于是；因此	1B
accredit /əˈkredɪt/	*vt.*	(of an official body) give authority or sanction to sb. or sth. when recognized standards have been met 认可；鉴定合格；委托，授权	7B
accredited /əˈkredɪtɪd/	*a.*	官方承认的	4L
accumulation /əˌkjuːmjuˈleɪʃ(ə)n/	*n.*	a mass or quantity of sth. that has gradually gathered or been acquired 积累；累积量	1B
acidosis /ˌæsɪˈdəusɪs/	*n.*	an excessively acid condition of the body fluids or tissues 酸中毒	7A
acquit /əˈkwɪt/	*vt.*	discharge (a duty or responsibility) 除去责任或义务	8A
acupuncture /ˈækjuˌpʌŋ(k)tʃə/	*n.*	a system of complementary medicine in which fine needles are inserted in the skin at specific points along what are considered to be lines of energy (meridians), used in the treatment of various physical and mental conditions 针刺	1A
acute /əˈkjuːt/	*a.*	(of a disease or its symptoms) severe but of short duration 急性的	3A
adaptive /əˈdæptɪv/	*a.*	characterized by or given to adaptation 适应的,有适应能力的	4B
adenosine /əˈdenə(u)siːn/	*n.*	a compound consisting of adenine（腺嘌呤）combined with ribose（核糖）, present in all living tissue in combined form as nucleotides 腺苷	6A
adept /əˈdept/	*a.*	very skilled or proficient at something 精于……的,擅长于……的	6A

220

adherence /ədˈhɪərəns/	n.	attachment or commitment to a person, cause, or belief 依附；坚持；忠诚	8B
adhesion /ədˈhiːʒən/	n.	an abnormal adhering of surfaces due to inflammation or injury 粘连	4B
adjunct /ˈædʒʌŋ(k)t/	a.	connected or added to sth., typically in an auxiliary way 附属的，辅助的	5B
administer /ədˈmɪnɪstə/	vt.	dispense or apply (a remedy or drug) 给予（病人药物）	5A
advocate /ˈædvəkət/	n.	a person who publicly supports or recommends a particular cause or policy 提倡者，拥护者	8B
aerobic /eəˈrəʊbɪk/	a.	relating to, involving, or requiring free oxygen 需氧的，有氧的	6A
affiliated /əˈfɪlɪeɪtɪd/	a.	(of a subsidiary group or a person) officially attached or connected to an organization 隶属的，附属的，有关联的	1A
affliction /əˈflɪkʃ(ə)n/	n.	a cause of pain or harm 苦恼，痛苦	6A
agent /ˈeɪdʒ(ə)nt/	n.	a substance that brings about a chemical or physical effect or causes a chemical reaction 任何能产生物理、化学或生物学效应的力、成分或物质；剂	1B
aggrandize /əˈgrændaɪz/	vt.	increase the power, status, or wealth of 增大，强化，扩大	8B
aggravate /ˈægrəveɪt/	vt.	to make an illness or a bad or unpleasant situation worse 加重，使恶化	5B
aggressive /əˈgresɪv/	a.	behaving or done in a determined and forceful way 积极进取的；有闯劲的；积极行动的	1B
agitation /ˌædʒɪˈteɪʃ(ə)n/	n.	a state of anxiety or nervous excitement 躁动	2A
ailment /ˈeɪlm(ə)nt/	n.	an illness, typically a minor one 疾病，小恙	7A
airway /ˈeəweɪ/	n.	气道	5L
albeit /ɔːlˈbiːɪt/	conj.	though 尽管，即使	7B
alienation /ˌeɪlɪəˈneɪʃ(ə)n/	n.	the act of making somebody less friendly or sympathetic towards you 离间，疏远	6A
allegation /ˌælɪˈgeɪʃ(ə)n/	n.	a claim or assertion that sb. has done sth. illegal or wrong, typically one made without proof 陈述，主张；指控	8B
allergen /ˈælədʒ(ə)n/	n.	a substance that causes an allergy 过敏原	
allergic /əˈlɜːdʒɪk/	a.	caused by or relating to an allergy 敏感的，过敏性的	7B
allergy /ˈælədʒi/	n.	变态反应，过敏	1L
alleviate /əˈliːvieɪt/	vt.	make (suffering, deficiency, or a problem) less severe 减轻，缓和	4A
alloy /ˈælɔɪ/	n.	a metal that is formed by mixing two types of metal together, or by mixing metal with another substance 合金	4A
amnesia /æmˈniːzɪə/	n.	a partial or total loss of memory 健忘症	5A
analgesia /ˌæn(ə)lˈdʒiːzɪə/	n.	the condition of being unable to feel pain while conscious 镇痛	7A
analgesic /ˌæn(ə)lˈdʒiːzɪk/	a.	(of a drug) acting to relieve pain 止痛的	4B

221

anatomic /ˌænəˈtɔmik/	*a.*	relating to bodily structure 解剖的	2A
anesthesia /ˌænɪsˈθiːzɪə/	*n.*	insensitivity to pain, especially as artificially induced by the administration of gases or the injection of drugs before surgical operations 麻醉	4A
antagonistic /æn,tæg(ə)ˈnɪstɪk/	*a.*	active opposition of hostility towards someone or sth. 敌对的,反对的	2B
antelope /ˈæntɪləup/	*n.*	a swift-running deer-like ruminant（反刍动物）with smooth hair and upward-pointing horns 羚羊	5A
anticholinergic /ˌæntɪˌkəulɪˈnəːdʒɪk/	*n.*	an anticholinergic drug 抗胆碱能药物	5A
anus /ˈeɪnəs/	*n.*	the opening at the end of the alimentary canal through which solid waste matter leaves the body 肛门	2A
aphasia /əˈfeɪzɪə/	*n.*	inability to understand or produce speech 失语	2B
appendectomy /ˌæp(ə)nˈdektəmi/	*n.*	a surgical operation to remove the appendix 阑尾切除术	7A
appendicitis /ə,pendəˈsaɪtɪs/	*n.*	阑尾炎	4L
applicable /əˈplɪkəb(ə)l/	*a.*	relevant or appropriate 适当的	3A
apprenticeship /əˈprentɪ(s)ʃɪp/	*n.*	employment as an apprentice 学徒工,当学徒;(中医)师承模式	1A
appropriate /əˈprəuprɪeɪt/	*vt.*	take (sth.) for one's own use, typically without the owner's permission 盗用;侵吞	8A
archaeological /ˌɑːkɪəˈlɒdʒɪk(ə)l/	*a.*	connected with the study of cultures of the past and of periods of history by examining the remains of buildings and objects found in the ground 考古学的,考古学上的	4A
artery /ˈɑːtəri/	*a.*	any of the tubes that carry blood from the heart to other parts of the body 动脉	3B
arthralgia /ɑːˈθrældʒə/	*n.*	pain in a joint 关节痛	4A
arthritis /ɑːˈθraɪtɪs/	*n.*	关节炎	1L
artifact /ˈɑːtɪfækt/	*n.*	an object made by a human being, typically one of cultural or historical interest 人工制品,手工艺品	6A
ascribe /əˈskraɪb/	*vi.*	regard sth. as being due to (a cause) 把……归于	2A
ashen /ˈæʃ(ə)n/	*a.*	(of a person's face) very pale with shock, fear, or illness 灰白色的	1B
asparagus /əˈspærəgəs/	*n.*	a tall plant of the lily family with fine feathery foliage（叶子）, cultivated for its edible shoots 芦笋	6B
aspirant /əˈspaɪərənt/	*n.*	有抱负的人	8L
assertive /əˈsəːtɪv/	*a.*	having or showing a confident and forceful personality 坚定而自信的	1B
assimilate /əˈsɪmɪleɪt/	*vt.*	absorb and digest 吸收,消化	2B
asthma /ˈæsmə/	*n.*	哮喘	1L
asthmatic /æsˈmætɪk/	*a.*	气喘的,哮喘病的	5L
asthmatic episode	*a.*	哮喘发作	5L

astringent /əˈstrɪn(d)ʒ(ə)nt/	a.	causing the contraction of skin cells and other body tissues 收涩的	2A
atherosclerosis /ˌæθərəuskliəˈrəusɪs/	n.	a disease of the arteries characterized by the deposition of fatty material on their inner walls 动脉粥样硬化	5A
atrial /ˈeɪtrɪəl/	a.	of or relating to an atrium 心房的	7A
attribute /ˈætrɪbjuːt/	n.	a quality or feature regarded as a characteristic or inherent part of sb. or sth. 品质，特征	6B
authentic /ɔːˈθentɪk/	a.	of undisputed origin and not a copy; genuine 真正的，真实的	6B
Ayurvedic /ˌɑːjuəˈveɪdɪk/	a.	related to the traditional Hindu system of medicine, which is based on the idea of balance in bodily systems and uses diet, herbal treatment, and yogic breathing 印度医学的	7B
backbone /ˈbækbəun/	n.	the chief support of a system or organization 中坚力量；骨干；支柱	1A
bedwetting /ˈbedwetɪŋ/	n.	involuntary urination during the night 尿床	5B
benevolent /bəˈnevələnt/	a.	仁慈的	8L
bequeath /bɪˈkwiːð/	vt.	pass sth. on or leave sth. to sb. else 将（财物等）遗赠给；将（知识等）传给（后人）	8A
bilateral /baɪˈlæt(ə)r(ə)l/	a.	having or relating to two sides 两侧的	5A
biomedicine /ˌbaɪəuˈmedsɪn/	n.	relating to both biology and medicine 生物医学	1A
bladder /ˈblædə/	n.	anything inflated and hollow 囊状物	3B
blockage /ˈblɒkɪdʒ/	n	an obstruction which makes movement or flow difficult or impossible 堵塞，阻滞	6A
bolster /ˈbəulstə/	vt.	support or strengthen 支持，支撑	6A
breathlessness /ˈbreθləsnəs/	n.	gasping for breath, typically due to exertion 喘不过气	3A
breech /briːtʃ/	n.	(archaic) a person's buttocks [古] 臀部	7A
bronchial /ˈbrɒŋkɪəl/	a.	支气管的	5L
bronchitis /brɒŋˈkaɪtɪs/	n.	支气管炎	5L
broncho-dilating /ˈbrɒŋkəu daɪˈleɪtɪŋ/	a.	related to the dilation of the bronchial tubes 扩张支气管的	5B
buttock /ˈbʌtək/	n.	either of the two round fleshy parts of the human body that form the bottom 臀部	4B
carbuncle /ˈkɑːbʌŋkl/	n.	a large painful swelling under the skin 痈	4A
categorization /ˌkætəgəraɪˈzeɪʃ(ə)n/	n.	编目方法，分门别类	6L
categorize /ˈkætəgəraɪz/	vt.	place in a particular class or group 把……归类，把……分门别类	6B
celery /ˈseləri/	n.	a cultivated plant of the parsley family, with closely packed succulent（多汁的）leaf stalks which are used as a salad or cooked vegetable 芹菜	6B
cerebral /ˈserɪbr(ə)l/	a.	relating to the brain 大脑的	5A

chaperone /ˈʃæpərəʊn/	n.	a person who accompanies and looks after another person or group of people 保护人；监护人	8B
charismatic /ˌkærɪzˈmætɪk/	a.	exercising a compelling charm which inspires devotion in others 有魅力的；神授的	8A
chemotherapy /ˌkiːmə(ʊ)ˈθerəpi/	n.	the treatment of disease by the use of chemical substances, especially the treatment of cancer by cytotoxic (细胞毒素的) and other drugs 化疗	7A
chop /tʃɔp/	vt.	cut (sth.) into pieces with repeated sharp blows of an axe or knife 切碎，砍	6B
chronic /ˈkrɔnɪk/	a.	慢性的；长期的	1L
cinnamon /ˈsɪnəmən/	n.	an aromatic spice made from the peeled, dried, and rolled bark of a SE Asian tree 樟属植物；桂皮香料	6B
circulation /ˌsəːkjʊˈleɪʃ(ə)n/	n.	血液循环	1L
circumscribe /ˈsəːkəmskraɪb/	vt.	restrict (sth.) within limits 限制；限定	1B
clash /klæʃ/	n.	冲突	7L
clinician /klɪˈnɪʃn/	n.	a doctor having direct contact with patients rather than being involved with theoretical or laboratory studies 临床医生	1B
clue /kluː/	n.	线索	3L
coagulation /kəʊˌægjuˈleɪʃn/	n.	the process of a liquid becoming thick and partly solid 凝结、凝血	4A
coexistence /ˌkəʊɪgˈzɪstəns/	n.	the state or fact of living or existing at the same time or in the same place 共存	3A
coincide /ˌkəʊɪnˈsaɪd/	vi.	occur at the same time 同时发生	3A
collaboration /kəˌlæbəˈreɪʃn/	n.	the action of working with sb. to produce sth. 合作，协作	7B
columnist /ˈkɔləmnɪst/	n.	专栏作家	4L
coma /ˈkəʊmə/	n.	a prolonged state of deep unconsciousness 昏迷	2B
commentator /ˈkɔmənteɪtə/	n.	a person who comments on events or on a text 注解者；评论员	8A
compassionate /kəmˈpæʃ(ə)nət/	a.	feeling or showing sympathy and concern for others 有同情心的；表示怜悯的	8B
complement /ˈkɔmplɪm(ə)nt/	n.	a thing that contributes extra features to sth. else in such a way as to improve or emphasize its quality 补足物	2A
complementary /ˌkɔmplɪˈment(ə)ri/	a.	combing in such a way as to enhance or emphasize the qualities of each other or another 互补的，补充的	2B
complexion /kəmˈplekʃ(ə)n/	n.	the natural color, texture, and appearance of a person's skin, especially of the face 面色；肤色	1B
complication /ˌkɔmplɪˈkeɪʃ(ə)n/	n.	并发症	5L
compress /ˈkɔmpres/	n.	a cloth that is pressed onto a part of the body to stop the loss of blood, reduce pain, etc. (用于退热、止血等的)敷布	1B
conductivity /ˌkɔndʌkˈtɪvəti/	n.	ability to conduct electricity, heat, etc. 传导性	4A

cone /kəʊn/	n.	a solid or hollow object with a round flat base and sides that slope up to a point 圆锥体	4A
confidentiality /ˌkɒnfɪˌdenʃɪˈælɪti/	n.	the state of keeping or being kept secret or private 机密性	8B
configuration /kənˌfɪgəˈreɪʃ(ə)n/	n.	an arrangement of the parts of sth. or a group of things结构, 构型,组态	1B
Confucianism /kənˈfjuːʃənɪz(ə)m/	n.	a system of philosophical and ethical teachings founded by Confucius and developed by Mencius 儒教,儒家学说	1A
congeal /kənˈdʒiːl/	vi.	become semi-solid, especially on cooling 凝结	3A
conscientiously /ˌkɒnʃɪˈenʃəsli/	ad.	in a way that is motivated by one's moral sense of right and wrong 凭良心地;认真负责地	8A
consciousness /ˈkɒnʃəsnɪs/	n.	the state of being aware of and responsive to one's surroundings 意识	2B
constipated /ˈkɒnstɪpeɪtɪd/	a.	unable to get rid of waste material from the bowels easily 患便秘的	1B
constitution /ˌkɒnstɪˈtjuːʃ(ə)n/	n.	a person's physical state as regards vitality, health, and strength 体质;体格	1B
constricted /kənˈstrɪktɪd/	a.	收缩的	5L
consultation /ˌkɒnsəlˈteɪʃ(ə)n/	n.	the action or process of formally consulting or discussing 咨询,请教	7B
containment /kənˈteɪnm(ə)nt/	n.	控制;抑制	2L
contraindicate /ˌkɒntrəˈɪndɪkeɪt/	vt.	advise against or indicate the possible danger of a drug, treatment, etc. 对……禁忌,（药物或疗法）禁用于	4A
convertible /kənˈvɜːtɪb(ə)l/	a.	able to be changed in form, function, or character 可改变的;可变换的	2A
convert /kənˈvɜːt/	vt.	change the form, character, or function of sth. 使转变	1A
convey /kənˈveɪ/	vt.	make (an idea, impression, or feeling) known or understandable 表达,传达	1A
coordination /kəʊˌɔːdɪˈneɪʃ(ə)n/	n.	the organization of the different elements of a complex body or activity so as to enable them to work together effectively 协调,和谐	2B
opioid /ˈəʊpɪˌɔɪd/	n.	阿片类药物	4L
copious /ˈkəʊpɪəs/	a.	abundant in supply or quantity 丰富的,大量的	2B
corrosive /kəˈrəʊsɪv/	a.	tending to destroy sth. slowly by chemical action 腐蚀性的	4A
counterbalance /ˈkaʊntəˌbæl(ə)ns/	vt.	neutralize or cancel by exerting an opposite influence 抵消	2A
courtesy /ˈkɜːtɪsi/	n.	the showing of politeness in one's attitude and behaviour towards others 谦恭有礼,礼貌	8B
credit /ˈkredɪt/	n.	public acknowledgement or praise, given or received when a person's responsibility for an action or idea becomes apparent 赞誉	1A
creed /kriːd/	n.	a system of religious belief; a faith（尤指宗教）信条,教义; 纲领	8B

criterion /kraɪˈtɪərɪən/	n.	(pl. criteria) a principle or standard by which sth. may be judged or decided 标准,规则	7B
crucial /ˈkruːʃ(ə)l/	a.	of great importance 关键性的	3A
cuisine /kwɪˈziːn/	n.	a style or method of cooking, especially as characteristic of a particular country, region, or establishment 烹饪;菜肴	6B
curriculum /kəˈrɪkjʊləm/	n.	(pl. curricula) the subjects comprising a course of study in a school or college 课程	7B
customize /ˈkʌstəmaɪz/	vt.	modify (sth.) to suit a particular individual or task 定制	5B
debilitation /dɪˌbɪlɪˈteɪʃ(ə)n/	n.	weakening and loss of energy 虚弱,无力,乏力	2B
deceptively /dɪˈseptɪvli/	ad.	in a way or to an extent that gives a misleading impression 迷惑地	3B
deduct /dɪˈdʌkt/	vt.	use the knowledge or information you have to understand sth. or form an opinion 演绎	1A
defect /ˈdiːfekt/	n.	a shortcoming, imperfection, or lack 瑕疵;欠缺,缺点	8A
deficiency /dɪˈfɪʃ(ə)nsi/	n.	a lack of shortage 缺乏,不足	2A
degeneration /dɪˌdʒenəˈreɪʃ(ə)n/	n.	deterioration and loss of function in the cells of a tissue or organ 退化,恶化	5A
degenerative /dɪˈdʒen(ə)rətɪv/	a.	退步的,变质的,退化的	1L
delegation /ˌdelɪˈgeɪʃn/	n.	a group of people who represent the views of an organization, a country, etc. 代表团	4A
deliberate /dɪˈlɪb(ə)rət/	a.	done consciously and intentionally 故意的;蓄意的	6A
delirious /dɪˈlɪrɪəs/	a.	in an acutely disturbed state of mind characterized by restlessness, illusion, and incoherence 精神错乱的,发狂的	2B
depict /dɪˈpɪkt/	vt.	portray in words; describe 描述	3B
depletion /dɪˈpliːʃn/	n.	reduction in the number or quantity of something 消耗,用尽,耗减	2B
dermatological /ˌdɜːmətəˈlɒdʒɪk(ə)l/	a.	pertaining to the branch of medicine concerned with the diagnosis and treatment of skin 皮肤病学的	7B
descend /dɪˈsend/	vi.	move or fall downwards 下降	3A
detective /dɪˈtektɪv/	n.	侦探	3L
detergent /dɪˈtɜːdʒ(ə)nt/	n.	a water-soluble cleansing agent which combines with impurities and dirt to make them more soluble, and differs from soap in not forming a scum（浮沫）with the salts in hard water 洗涤剂;去垢剂	6B
devoid /dɪˈvɔɪd/	a.	entirely lacking or free from 缺乏,没有	8B
dexterously /ˈdekstrəsli/	ad.	in a way that shows the ability to perform a difficult action quickly and skillfully with the hands 灵巧地	4A
diabetes /daɪəˈbiːtiːz/	n.	糖尿病	3L
diagnosis /ˌdaɪəgˈnəʊsɪs/	n.	the identification of the nature of an illness or other problem by examination of the symptoms 诊断	1A
diaphoresis /ˌdaɪəfəˈriːsɪs/	n.	sweating, especially to an unusual degree as a symptom of disease or a side effect of a drug 发汗	1A

diarrhea /ˌdaɪəˈrɪə/	*n.*	an illness in which waste matter is emptied from the bowels much more frequently than normal, and in liquid form 腹泻	4A
dice /daɪs/	*vt.*	cut (food or other matter) into small cubes 将……切成丁	6B
dictate /dɪkˈteɪt/	*vt.*	control or decisively affect; determine 支配，决定	4B
dietary /ˈdaɪət(ə)ri/	*a.*	relating to or provided by diet 饮食的，规定食物的	1A
differentiation /ˌdɪfərenʃɪˈeɪʃn/	*n.*	the action or process of differentiating 辨别	1A
digestion /daɪˈdʒestʃ(ə)n/	*n.*	a person's capacity to digest food 消化	3B
diminish /dɪˈmɪnɪʃ/	*vi.*	make or become less 减弱，减轻	1B
discern /dɪˈsɜːn/	*vt.*	recognize or find out 看出；理解，了解	1B
discharge /dɪsˈtʃɑːdʒ/	*v.*	allow (a liquid, gas, or other substance) to flow out from where it has been confined 排放	2A
discipline /ˈdɪsɪplɪn/	*n.*	a branch of knowledge, typically one studied in higher education 学科	6A
discretion /dɪˈskreʃ(ə)n/	*n.*	the quality of behaving or speaking in such a way as to avoid causing offence or revealing confidential information 慎重；考虑周到；判断力，辨别力	8A
disenchantment /ˌdɪs(ɪ)nˈtʃɑːntm(ə)nt/	*n.*	a feeling of disappointment about sb. or sth. you previously respected or admired; disillusionment 觉醒，清醒	6A
disreputable /dɪsˈrepjʊtəb(ə)l/	*a.*	not considered to be respectable in character or appearance 名誉不好的，不体面的	8A
disruption /dɪsˈrʌpʃn/	*n.*	紊乱，失调	1L
dissipate /ˈdɪsɪpeɪt/	*vt.*	disperse or scatter 驱散	2A
distention /dɪsˈtenʃən/	*n.*	the state of being stretched beyond normal dimensions 膨胀；延伸	4A
distress /dɪˈstres/	*vt.*	cause (someone) anxiety, sorrow, or pain 使痛苦	3A
divert /daɪˈvɜːt/	*vt.*	cause sb. or sth. to change course or turn from one direction to another 使……改道，转向	8A
dogma /ˈdɒgmə/	*n.*	a principle or set of principles laid down by an authority as incontrovertibly true 教义，教条，信条	8A
dominant /ˈdɒmɪnənt/	*a.*	having power and influence over others 占优势的；占支配地位的	4A
dopamine /ˈdəʊpəmiːn/	*n.*	a compound present in the body as a neurotransmitter and a precursor of other substances including adrenaline 多巴胺	7A
dopaminergic /ˌdəʊpəmɪˈnɜːdʒɪk/	*a.*	releasing or involving dopamine as a neurotransmitter 多巴胺能的	5A
downbearing /daʊnˈbeərɪŋ/	*n.*	turning and proceeding in a downward direction 向下	2A
drainage /ˈdreɪnɪdʒ/	*n.*	the action or process of draining sth. 排水	2A
dredge /dredʒ/	*vt.*	clear the bed of (a harbor, river, or other area of water) by scooping out mud, weeds, and rubbish with a dredge 疏通，清淤(河道等)	4A

dressing /ˈdresɪŋ/	n.	a piece of material used to cover and protect a wound 敷料	7A
duality /djuːˈælɪti/	n.	二元性	2L
durable /ˈdjʊərəb(ə)l/	a.	likely to last for a long time without breaking or getting weaker 耐用的	4A
dysentery /ˈdɪsəntri/	n.	an infection of the bowels that causes severe diarrhea with loss of blood 痢疾	4A
dysmenorrhea /ˌdɪsmenəˈriːə/	n.	painful menstruation, typically involving abdominal cramps 痛经	3A
edema /ɪˈdiːmə/	n.	a condition characterized by an excess of watery fluid collecting in the cavities or tissues of the body 水肿	3A
effuse /ɪˈfjuːs/	vt.	give off (a liquid, light, smell, or quality) 涌出, 流出	2A
elastic /ɪˈlæstɪk/	a.	able to stretch and return to its original 有弹性的	4A
electrostimulation /iˌlektrəˌstimjuˈleiʃ ən/	n.	electrical stimulation of a nerve, muscle, etc. 电刺激	4A
eliminate /ɪˈlɪmɪneɪt/	vt.	expel (waste matter) from the body 消除	3A
embolism /ˈembəlɪz(ə)m/	n.	obstruction of an artery, typically by a clot of blood or an air bubble 栓塞	7A
emetic /ɪˈmetɪk/	a.	(of a substance) causing vomiting 催吐的	1A
emphysema /ˌemfɪˈsiːmə/	n.	a condition in which the air sacs of the lungs are damaged and enlarged, causing breathlessness 肺气肿	7A
encompass /ɪnˈkʌmpəs/	vt.	include comprehensively 包含, 包括	1A
endeavor /ɪnˈdevə/	n.	an attempt to achieve a goal 努力, 尽力	6A
endocrine /ˈendə(ʊ)kraɪn/	a.	relating to or denoting glands which secrete hormones or other products directly into the blood 内分泌(腺)的, 激素的	1B
endoscopy /enˈdɒskəpi/	n.	a procedure in which an instrument is introduced into the body to give a view of its internal parts 内镜检查术	1B
energize /ˈenədʒaɪz/	vt.	给……以活力, 使活跃	6L
entity /ˈentɪti/	n.	a thing with distinct and independent existence 独立存在体; 实体	1B
entrust /ɪnˈtrʌst/	vt.	assign the responsibility for doing sth. to sb. 委托, 托付	8A
epidemic /ˌepɪˈdemɪk/	a.	(of a disease) with large numbers of cases occurring at the same time in a particular community 流行性的	1A
epigastric /ˌepɪˈgæstrɪk/	a.	of or relating to the anterior walls of the abdomen 胃脘部的, 上腹部的	4A
episode /ˈepɪsəʊd/	n.	a finite period in which sb. is affected by a specified illness (某疾病) 的发作期	5B
equilibrium /ˌiːkwɪˈlɪbrɪəm/	n.	a state in which opposing forces or influences are balanced 平衡	6A
eradicate /ɪˈrædɪkeɪt/	vt.	destroy completely; put an end to 摧毁; 完全根除	6A
exactitude /ɪgˈzæktɪtjuːd/	n.	the quality of being exact 正确; 严谨	8A

excess /ɪkˈses/	n.	an amount of sth. that is more than necessary, permitted, or desirable 超过	2A
exertion /ɪgˈzɜːʃn/	n.	physical or mental effort 努力，费力 abundant in supply or quantity 丰富的；很多的	5B
exhort /ɪgˈzɔːt/	vt.	strongly encourage or urge sb. to do sth. 劝告，劝说；倡导	8B
expertise /ˌekspɜːˈtiːz/	n.	expert skill or knowledge in a particular field 专业知识或技能	1A
exposure /ɪkˈspəʊʒə/	n.	the state of having no protection from contact with sth. harmful 暴露	5B
extensive /ɪkˈstensɪv/	a.	large in amount or scale 大量的	1B
exterior /ɪkˈstɪərɪə/	a.	forming, situated on, or relating to the outside of sth. 外部的	3A
extinguish /ɪkˈstɪŋgwɪʃ/	vt.	cause (a fire or light) to cease to burn or shine 熄灭（火）	1B
extremity /ɪkˈstremɪti/	n.	the hands and feet 肢体	2B
exuberance /egˈz(j)uːb(ə)r(ə)ns/	n.	the quality of being full of energy, excitement, and cheerfulness 丰富，充沛，充盈	2B
facilitate /fəˈsɪlɪteɪt/	vt.	make (an action or process) easy or easier 促进，助长；帮助	8B
facility /fəˈsɪlɪti/	n.	a place, amenity, or piece of equipment provided for a particular purpose 设施，设备	7B
fad /fæd/	n.	an intense and widely shared enthusiasm for sth., especially one that is short-lived; a craze 一时的流行；一时的风尚	8A
fallacy /ˈfæləsi/	n.	a mistaken belief, especially one based on unsound arguments 谬误，谬论	6A
fatigue /fəˈtiːg/	n.	疲倦	4L
febrile /ˈfiːbraɪl/	a.	having or showing the symptoms of a fever 发热的	1A
feeble-mindedness /ˌfiːb(ə)lˈmaɪndɪdnəs/	n.	having less than average intelligence 低能，愚痴	2B
fetal /ˈfiːt(ə)l/	a.	relating to a fetus 胎儿的	7A
fetus /ˈfiːtəs/	n.	an unborn offspring of a mammal, in particular an unborn human baby more than eight weeks after conception 胎儿	3B
fiberscope /ˈfaɪbəˌskəʊp/	n.	a fiber-optic device for viewing inaccessible internal structures, especially in the human body 纤维镜	1B
fibromyalgia /ˌfaɪbrəʊmaɪˈældʒɪə/	n.	a rheumatic condition characterized by muscular or musculoskeletal pain with stiffness and localized tenderness at specific points on the body 纤维性肌痛	7A
fibrosis /faɪˈbrəʊsɪs/	n.	the thickening and scarring of connective tissue, usually as a result of injury 纤维化	7A
fidgety /ˈfɪdʒɪti/	a.	restless or uneasy 坐立不安的；烦躁的	1B
filiform /ˈfaɪlɪfɔːm/	a.	thread-like 丝状的；线状的；纤维状的	4A
flick /flɪk/	vt.	hit sth. with a sudden quick movement, especially using your finger and thumb together, or your hand 轻弹；轻拍	4A
fluidity /fluːˈɪdɪti/	n.	流动性；不稳定	2L

flux /flʌks/	n.	the action or process of flowing or flowing out 流量,流出	2A
formula /ˈfɔːmjulə/	n.	配方,处方;方剂(中医学)	1L
fortify /ˈfɔːtɪfaɪ/	vt.	strengthen 增强	5B
foster /ˈfɒstə/	vt.	encourage the development of (sth., especially sth. desirable) 培养;促进	6A
fraudulent /ˈfrɔːdjʊl(ə)nt/	a.	obtained, done by, or involving deception, especially criminal deception 欺骗的,不诚实的;奸诈的	8A
frigidity /frɪˈdʒɪdɪti/	n.	(in a woman) the lack of the ability to enjoy sex(尤指妇女的)性感缺失,性冷淡	6A
gait /geɪt/	n.	a person's manner of walking 步态	5A
gall /gɔːl/	n.	bile 胆汁	3B
garlic /ˈgɑːlɪk/	n.	a strong-smelling pungent-tasting bulb, used as flavoring in cooking and in herbal medicine 大蒜;蒜头	6B
gastritis /gæˈstraɪtɪs/	n.	inflammation of the lining of the stomach 胃炎	6A
gastrointestinal /ˌgæstrəʊɪnˈtestɪn(ə)l/	a.	of or relating to the stomach and the intestines 胃肠的	1B
gauze /gɔːz/	n.	a type of thin cotton cloth used for covering and protecting wounds 纱布	4A
generate /ˈdʒenəreɪt/	vt.	产生,引起	2L
genetics /dʒəˈnetɪks/	n.	the qualities and characteristics passed from each generation of living things to the next 遗传,遗传特征	5B
ginger /ˈdʒɪndʒə/	n.	a hot, fragrant spice made from the rhizome(根茎)of a plant, which may be chopped or powdered for cooking, preserved in syrup, or candied 生姜	6B
greasy /ˈgriːsi/	a.	covered with, resembling, or produced by grease or oil 油腻的	4B
groan /grəʊn/	n.	the action or state of making a deep inarticulate sound in response to pain or despair 呻吟	3B
guanosine /ˈgwɑːnəsiːn/	n.	a compound consisting of guanine combined with ribose, present in all living tissue in combined form as nucleotides 鸟苷,鸟嘌呤核苷	6A
gynecological /ˌgaɪnəkəˈlɒdʒikəl/	a.	妇科的	4L
heed /hiːd/	vt.	pay attention to; take notice of 注意,留心	1B
heighten /ˈhaɪt(ə)n/	vt.	make or become more intense(使)变高,(使)加强	6A
herbal /ˈhəːb(ə)l/	a.	relating to or made from herbs, especially those used in cooking and medicine 药草的,草本的	1A
hernia /ˈhəːnɪə/	n.	a condition in which part of an organ is displaced and protrudes through the wall of the cavity containing it 疝气	7A
highlight /ˈhaɪlaɪt/	vt.	强调,突出	2L
holistic /həʊˈlɪstɪk/	a.	characterized by the treatment of the whole person, taking into account mental and social factors, rather than just the symptoms of a disease 整体的	1A

holographic /ˌhɒləˈɡræfɪk/	*a.*	produced using holograms 全息的	3B
humanitarian /hjuːˌmænɪˈteːrɪən/	*a.*	concerned with or seeking to promote human welfare 人道主义的；博爱的	8B
	n.	a person who seeks to promote human welfare 人道主义者；博爱主义者	
hypokinesis /ˌhaipəʊkɪˈniːsɪs/	*n.*	decreased bodily movement 运动减退	5A
iconic /aɪˈkɒnɪk/	*a.*	of the nature of an icon 符号的，图标的	3B
ignite /ɪɡˈnaɪt/	*vt.*	cause to catch fire 点燃	4A
illegal /ɪˈliːɡ(ə)l/	*a.*	非法的，不合法的	7L
immunity /ɪˈmjuːnɪti/	*n.*	免疫力	2L
imperative /ɪmˈperətɪv/	*a.*	of vital importance; crucial 极重要的；必要的	1A
impermanence /ɪmˈpəːmənəns/	*n.*	暂时，无常	2L
implicitly /ɪmˈplɪsɪtli/	*ad.*	with no qualification or question, absolutely 无条件地，绝对地，无疑问地	8B
impose /ɪmˈpəʊz/	*vt.*	强加，强迫	7L
impotence /ˈɪmpət(ə)ns/	*n.*	inability in a man to achieve an erection or orgasm 阳痿	6A
incidence /ˈɪnsɪd(ə)ns/	*n.*	the occurrence, rate, or frequency of a disease, crime, or other undesirable thing 发生率	5B
incoherent /ˌɪnkə(ʊ)ˈhɪər(ə)nt/	*a.*	not logical or internally consistent 前后矛盾的，不一致的	1A
incorporate /ɪnˈkɔːpəreɪt/	*vt.*	包含；吸收；合并	1L
index /ˈɪndeks/ (finger)	*n.*	the finger next to the thumb 食指	4A
indigestion /ˌɪndɪˈdʒestʃən/	*n.*	消化不良	4L
indissolubly /ˌɪndɪˈsɒljʊbli/	*ad.*	in a way that is unable to be destroyed, undone, or broken 不可分解地	3A
induce /ɪnˈdjuːs/	*vt.*	bring about or give rise to 引起；导致	1A
induct /ɪnˈdʌkt/	*vt.*	use known facts to produce rules or principles 归纳	1A
induction /ɪnˈdʌkʃ(ə)n/	*n.*	the action or process of bringing about or giving rise to sth. 诱发	7A
infectious /ɪnˈfekʃəs/	*a.*	(of a disease or disease-causing organism) liable to be transmitted to people, organism, etc. through the environment 传染的；有传染性的	1A
infertility /ˌɪnfəˈtɪlɪti/	*n.*	inability to conceive children or young 不孕	4L
inflammation /ˌɪnfləˈmeɪʃn/	*n.*	a localized physical condition in which part of the body becomes reddened, swollen, hot, and often painful, especially as a reaction to injury or infection 炎症，发炎	7A
ingredient /ɪnˈɡriːdɪənt/	*n.*	any of the foods or substances that are combined to make a particular dish（烹调的）原料	6B
ingredient /ɪnˈɡriːdɪənt/	*n.*	one of the things from which sth. is made 成分，组成部分	5B
inhale /ɪnˈheɪl/	*vt.*	breathe in 吸入	5B
inhaler /ɪnˈheɪlə/	*n.*	吸入器	5L
inherently /ɪnˈhɪərəntli/	*ad.*	in a permanent, essential, or characteristic way 天性地，固有地	8A

initial /ɪ'nɪʃl/	a.	happening at the beginning 最初的	4A
Inner Mongolia /mɔŋ'ɡəʊliə/	n.	an autonomous region of northeast China 内蒙古	4A
insert /ɪn'sɜːt/	vt.	put sth. into sth. else 插入	4A
insomnia /ɪn'sɔmnɪə/	n.	habitual sleeplessness; inability to sleep 失眠，失眠症	1B
instinctively /ɪn'stɪŋktɪvli/	ad.	without conscious thought; by natural instinct 本能地	4A
integrate /'ɪntɪɡreɪt/	vt.	combine (one thing) with another to form a whole 使整合	3B
integration /ˌɪntɪ'ɡreɪʃ(ə)n/	n.	the act or process of combining two or more things so that they work together 结合，整合	6A
intensity /ɪn'tensɪti/	n.	the quality of being intense 强度	5A
interaction /ˌɪntər'ækʃ(ə)n/	n.	相互作用	2L
interior /ɪn'tɪərɪə/	a.	situated on or relating to the inside of sth. 内部的	3A
intermittent /ˌɪntə'mɪtənt/	a.	间歇的	4L
internship /'ɪntəːnʃɪp/	n.	the position of a student or trainee who works in an organization, sometimes without pay, in order to gain work experience or satisfy requirements for a qualification（美）实习医师，实习医师期	8A
intimately /'ɪntɪmətli/	ad.	熟悉地；亲密地	6L
intravenous /ˌɪntrə'viːnəs/	a.	existing or taking place within, or administered into, a vein or veins 静脉的，静脉注射的	7A
intricately /'ɪntrɪkətli/	ad.	in a very complicated or detailed manner 盘根错节地	2B
invasion /ɪn'veɪʒ(ə)n/	n.	an incursion（侵入）by a large number of people or things into a place or sphere of activity 侵袭	3A
isolable /'aɪsələb(ə)l/	a.	being in the state of identifying sth. and examine or deal with it separately 孤立的	1B
isometrics /ˌaɪsə(ʊ)'metrɪks/	n.	(pl.) a system of physical exercises in which muscles are caused to act against each other or against a fixed object 静力锻炼法	6A
isotonics /ˌaɪsə(ʊ)'tɔnɪks/	n.	muscular exercise using free weights or fixed devices to simulate resistance of weight 等张（力）训练	6A
jerky /'dʒəːki/	a.	characterized by abrupt stops and starts 忽动忽停的	4B
kinesiology /kɪˌniːsɪ'ɔlədʒi/	n.	the study of the mechanics of body movements 人体运动学	7A
knuckle /'nʌk(ə)l/	n.	part of a finger at a joint where the bone is near the surface, especially where the finger joins the hand 指关节	4B
lactate /'læpkteɪt/	n.	a salt or ester of lactic acid 乳酸	6A
lassitude /'læsɪtjuːd/	n.	a state of physical or mental weariness; lack of energy 懒怠	2B
layer /'leɪə/	vt.	arrange in a layer or layers 把……分层堆放	3B
legislation /ˌledʒɪs'leɪʃ(ə)n/	n.	the process of making or enacting laws 立法，制定法律	8B
lemonade /ˌlemə'neɪd/	n.	a drink made from lemon juice and water sweetened with sugar 柠檬汽水，柠檬饮料	6B

license /ˈlaɪs(ə)ns/	*vt.*	同意，发许可证	3L
lubricate /ˈluːbrɪkeɪt/	*vt.*	apply a substance such as oil or grease to (an engine or component) so as to minimize friction and allow smooth movement 使润滑	4B
lumbar /ˈlʌmbə/	*a.*	relating to the lower part of the back 腰部的	7A
lumbosacral /ˌlʌmbəʊˈseɪkrəl/	*a.*	of or relating to or near the small of the back and the back part of the pelvis between the hips 腰骶的	4A
lunge /lʌn(d)ʒ/	*n.*	the basic attacking move in fencing, in which the leading foot is thrust forward close to the floor with the knee bent while the back leg remains straightened 前腿弯曲后腿蹬直的弓箭步（击剑）	4B
lusterless /ˈlʌstələs/	*a.*	not bright or shiny 没有光泽的	2B
lustrous /ˈlʌstrəs/	*a.*	having luster, shining 光亮的，有光泽的	2B
macro /ˈmækrəʊ/	*a.*	large-scale; overall 宏观的；全面的	1A
macrocosm /ˈmækrə(ʊ)kɒz(ə)m/	*n.*	the whole of a complex structure, especially the world or the universe, contrasted with a small or representative part of it 宏观世界	3B
mainstay /ˈmeɪnsteɪ/	*n.*	sth. on which sth. else is based or relies 主要支柱	6A
malady /ˈmælədi/	*n.*	a disease or ailment 疾病，病症	6A
mammary /ˈmæməri/	*a.*	connected with the breasts 乳房的；乳腺的	4A
maneuver /məˈnuvə/	*n.*	a movement performed with care and skill 谨慎而熟练的动作	4A
manic /ˈmænɪk/	*a.*	relating to or affected by mania 躁狂的，患躁狂病的	2B
manifestation /ˌmænɪfeˈsteɪʃ(ə)n/	*n.*	a symptom of an ailment 表现，表现形式	1A
manipulation /məˌnɪpjʊˈleɪʃ(ə)n/	*n.*	the action of manipulating sth. in a skillful manner（熟练的）操作，操纵	4A
manufactory /ˌmænjʊˈfækt(ə)ri/	*n.*	制造厂，工厂	7L
maxim /ˈmæksɪm/	*n.*	箴言；格言	8L
mean /miːn/	*n.*	a condition, quality, or course of action equally removed from two opposite extremes 中间值，平均值	1A
medicinal /məˈdɪsɪn(ə)l/	*a.*	(of a substance or plant) having healing properties 医学的，药用的	2A
	n.	a medicinal substance 药品	
meditation /ˌmedɪˈteɪʃ(ə)n/	*n.*	the practice of thinking deeply in silence, especially for religious reasons or in order to make your mind calm 沉思，冥想	6A
melon /ˈmelən/	*n.*	the large round fruit of a plant of the gourd family, with sweet pulpy flesh and many seeds 甜瓜	6B
menstrual /ˈmenstruəl/	*a.*	relating to the menses or menstruation 月经的	3A
meridian /məˈrɪdɪən/	*n.*	（中医学）经，经络	1L
metabolic /ˌmetəˈbɒlɪk/	*a.*	新陈代谢的	1L

metallurgy /mə'tælədʒi/	n.	the scientific study of metals and their uses 冶金学；冶金术	4A
methodology /ˌmeθə'dɒlədʒi/	n.	a system of methods used in a particular area of study or activity（从事某一活动的）一套方法；方法论；方法学	1A
metropolitan /ˌmetrə'pɒlɪt(ə)n/	a.	connected with a large or capital city 大都会的，大城市的	6A
microcosm /'maɪkrə(ʊ)kɒz(ə)m/	n.	a community, place, or situation regarded as encapsulating in miniature the characteristics of sth. much larger 微观世界	3B
migraine /'miːɡreɪn/	n.	a recurrent throbbing headache that typically affects one side of the head and is often accompanied by nausea and disturbed vision 偏头痛	7B
miniature /'mɪnɪtʃə/	a.	very small of its kind 微小的，微型的	5B
minimize /'mɪnɪmaɪz/	vt.	将……减到最少	5L
miscellaneous /ˌmɪsə'leɪnɪəs/	a.	(of items or people gathered or considered together) of various types or from different sources 各种各样的；混杂的	1A
mite /maɪt/	n.	螨虫	5L
modality /mə(ʊ)'dælɪti/	n.	a method of therapy that involves physical or electrical therapeutic treatment　治疗方法	1A
moderation /ˌmɒdə'reɪʃ(ə)n/	n.	the avoidance of excess or extremes, especially in one's behavior or political opinions 温和，适度	2A
moisture /'mɔɪstʃə/	n.	water or other liquid diffused in a small quantity as vapor, within a solid, or condensed on a surface 水分；潮湿	3B
mold /məʊld/	n.	霉菌	5L
molestation /ˌməʊle'steɪʃ(ə)n/	n.	sexual assault or abuse of a person, especially a woman or child 骚扰	8B
monitor/'mɒnɪtə/	vt.	observe and check the progress or quality of (sth.) over a period of time 监控	5A
monograph /'mɒnəɡrɑːf/	n.	a detailed written study of a single specialized subject or an aspect of it 专著，专论	1A
monophosphate /ˌmɒnə'fɒsfeɪt/	n.	a chemical composition that only has one phosphate group 一磷酸盐	6A
morbidity /mɔː'bɪdɪti/	n.	the condition of being diseased 病态；发病	2A
moss /mɒs/	n.	a very small green or yellow plant without flowers that spreads over damp surfaces, rocks, trees, etc. 苔藓	1B
moxa /'mɒksə/	n.	a soft woolly mass prepared from the ground young leaves of a Eurasian Artemisia 艾	4A
moxibustion /ˌmɒksɪ'bʌstʃ(ə)n/	n.	the burning of moxa on or near a person's skin as a counterirritant 艾灸	1A
mugwort /'mʌɡwəːt/	n.	a plant of the daisy family, with aromatic divided leaves that are dark green above and whitish below, native to north temperate regions 艾蒿	4A
musculo-skeletal /ˌmʌskjʊləʊ 'skelətl/	a.	肌肉骨骼的	6L

mutual /ˈmjuːtʃ(ə)l/	a.	a feeling or action experienced or done by each of two or more parties towards the other or others 相互的，共有的	2B
naive /nɑːˈiːv/	a.	(of a person) natural and unaffected 天真的，单纯的	1A
narcotic /nɑːˈkɒtɪk/	n.	a drug which induces drowsiness, stupor, or insensibility, and relieves pain 麻醉药，镇静剂	7A
navel /ˈneɪv(ə)l/	n.	a rounded, knotty depression in the center of a person's belly caused by the detachment of the umbilical（脐带的）cord after birth 脐	3B
neo-confucianism /ˈniːəʊ kənˈfjuːʃənɪzm/	n.	理学	8L
Neolithic /ˌniːəˈlɪθɪk/	a.	of the latter part of the Stone Age 新石器时代的	4A
neuroanatomy /ˌnjʊərəʊəˈnætəmi/	n.	the anatomy of the nervous system 神经解剖学	7A
neuron /ˈnjʊərɒn/	n.	a specialized cell transmitting nerve impulses; a nerve cell 神经元	5A
norepinephrine /ˌnɔːrepɪˈnefriːn/	n.	a hormone which is released by the adrenal medulla and by the sympathetic nerves and functions as a neurotransmitter 去甲肾上腺素	7A
nourishment /ˈnʌrɪʃm(ə)nt/	n.	the food necessary for growth, health, and good condition 食物，营养物	2B
numbness /ˈnʌmnəs/	n.	a lack of feeling in a part of the body 无感觉；麻木	4A
nurture /ˈnɜːtʃə/	vt.	care for and protect sb. or sth. while they are growing 养育；培育	8B
nutmeg /ˈnʌtmeg/	n.	the hard, aromatic, almost spherical seed of a tropical tree 肉豆蔻	6B
odor /ˈəʊdə/	n.	a distinctive smell, especially an unpleasant one 气味	3B
olive /ˈɒlɪv/	n.	a small green or black fruit with a strong taste, used in cooking and for its oil 橄榄	4A
onset /ˈɒnset/	n.	the beginning of sth., especially sth. unpleasant 开始	6A
ontologically /ˌɒntəˈlɒdʒɪk(ə)li/	ad.	connected with the branch of philosophy that deals with the nature of existence 存在论地；本体论地	1B
optimum /ˈɒptɪməm/	a.	most conducive to a favorable outcome; best 最适宜的，最佳的	4B
organismic /ˌɔːg(ə)ˈnɪz(ə)mɪk/	a.	having the nature of, relating to or belonging to an organism (considered as a whole) 有机体的	1B
oriental /ˌɔːriˈent(ə)l/	a.	东方的；东方人的	6L
orthodox /ˈɔːθədɒks/	a.	following or conforming to the traditional or generally accepted rules or beliefs of a religion, philosophy, or practice 规范的；正统的	6A
outrage /ˈaʊtreɪdʒ/	n.	an extremely strong reaction of anger, shock, or indignation 义愤；愤慨	8B
overrate /ˌəʊvəˈreɪt/	vt.	have a higher opinion of (sb. or sth.) than is deserved 高估；评价过高	7A

oversee /ˌəʊvəˈsiː/	vt.	supervise (a person or their work), especially in an official capacity 监管，监督	7B
pad /pæd/	n.	a thick piece of soft material that is used, for example, for absorbing liquid, cleaning or protecting sth. 软垫	4A
painkiller /ˈpeɪnkɪlə/	n.	止痛药	4L
palpation /ˌpælˈpeɪʃ(ə)n/	n.	examining (a part of the body) by touch, especially for medical purposes 触诊，按诊	1B
palpitation /ˌpælpɪˈteɪʃ(ə)n/	n.	a noticeably rapid, strong, or irregular heartbeat due to agitation, exertion, or illness 心悸	2B
pancreas /ˈpæŋkrɪəs/	n.	胰，胰腺	6L
pandemic /pænˈdemɪk/	n.	大流行病	4A
pant /pænt/	vi.	breathe with short, quick breaths, typically from exertion or excitement 喘息	5B
papilla /pəˈpɪlə/	n.	(pl. papillae) a small rounded protuberance（突起）on a part or organ of the body 乳头	3B
papillae /pəˈpɪli/	n.	a small nipple-shaped protuberance 乳头状突起	4A
paralysis /pəˈrælɪsɪs/	n.	the loss of the ability to move (and sometimes to feel anything) in part or most of the body, typically as a result of illness, poison, or injury 瘫痪，麻痹	4B
parameter /pəˈræmɪtə/	n.	a numerical or other measurable factor forming one of a set that defines a system or sets the conditions of its operation 参数	2A
parasympathetic /ˌpærəˌsɪmpəˈθetɪk/	a..	副交感神经的	5L
pathogen /ˈpæθədʒ(ə)n/	n.	a bacterium, virus, or other microorganism that can cause disease 病原体	2A
pathogenic /ˌpæθəˈdʒænɪk/	a.	(of a bacterium, virus, or other microorganism) causing disease（细菌、病毒或其他微生物）病原的，致病的	1A
pathological /ˌpæθəˈlɒdʒɪk(ə)l/	a.	relating to pathology 病理学的	1B
pectoral /ˈpekt(ə)r(ə)l/	a.	relating to the breast or chest 胸部的	4B
pediatric /piːdɪˈætrɪk/	a.	relating to the branch of medicine dealing with children and their diseases 儿科的	5B
penetrate /ˈpenɪtreɪt/	vt.	go into or through (sth.), especially with force or effort 穿透	3B
peptic /ˈpeptɪk/	a.	of or relating to digestion, especially that in which pepsin （胃蛋白酶）is concerned 消化性的，（尤涉及）胃蛋白酶的	1B
perceive /pəˈsiːv/	vt.	become aware or conscious of sth.; come to realize or understand 意识到；理解	1B
perceptible /pəˈseptɪb(ə)l/	a.	(especially of a slight movement or change of state) able to be seen or noticed 可感觉（感受）到的，可理解的，可认识的	1B
perception /pəˈsepʃ(ə)n/	n.	the way in which sth. is regarded, understood, or interpreted 看法，理解，认识	1B

period /ˈpɪərɪəd/	*n.*	(also menstrual period) a flow of blood and other material from the lining of the uterus, lasting for a few days and occurring in sexually mature women who are not pregnant at intervals of about one lunar month until the menopause 月经	3A
perpendicular /ˌpɜːpənˈdɪkjələ/	*a.*	forming an angle of 90° with another line or surface 垂直的	4A
perpetuate /pəˈpetʃʊeɪt/	*vt.*	make (sth.) continue indefinitely 保持	3A
perspective /pəˈspektɪv/	*n.*	a particular attitude towards or way of regarding sth.; a point of view 看法, 观点	1B
perspiration /ˌpəːspɪˈreɪʃ(ə)n/	*n.*	the process of sweating 出汗, 流汗	2B
pharmacopeia /ˌfɑːməkəˈpiːə/	*n.*	处方汇编, 药典	6L
phlegm /flem/	*n.*	the thick viscous substance secreted by the mucous membranes of the respiratory passages, especially when produced in excessive quantities during a cold 痰	3A
physician /fɪˈzɪʃ(ə)n/	*n.*	a person qualified to practice medicine, especially one who specializes in diagnosis and medical treatment as distinct from surgery 医生;(尤指)内科医生	1B
physiological /ˌfɪzɪəˈlɒdʒɪk(ə)l/	*a.*	relating to the branch of biology that deals with the normal functions of living organisms and their parts 生理的	1B
physiotherapy /ˌfɪzɪə(ʊ)ˈθerəpi/	*n.*	the treatment of disease, injury, or deformity by physical methods such as massage, heat treatment, and exercise rather than by drugs or surgery 理疗	7B
pinpoint /ˈpɪnpɔɪnt/	*vt.*	find or identify with great accuracy or precision 确定, 精准定位	3B
pit /pɪt/	*n.*	the large hard seed of a fruit or vegetable 核	4A
pivotal /ˈpɪvətl/	*a.*	fixed on or as if on a pivot 枢轴的	4B
pleurisy /ˈplʊərɪsi/	*n.*	inflammation of the pleurae, which impairs their lubricating function and causes pain when breathing, causing by pneumonia and other diseases of the chest or abdomen 胸膜炎	7A
plunder /ˈplʌndə/	*vt.*	take material from (artistic or academic work) for one's own purposes 取用	3B
pneumonectomy /ˌnjuːmə(ʊ)ˈnektəmɪ/	*n.*	surgical removal of a lung or part of a lung 肺切除术	4A
pneumonia /njuːˈməʊnɪə/	*n.*	lung inflammation caused by bacterial or viral infection 肺炎	1B
pollen /ˈpɒlən/	*n.*	花粉	5L
porous /ˈpɔːrəs/	*a.*	(of a rock or other material) having minute interstices through which liquid or air may pass 能穿透的, 能渗透的; 有毛孔或气孔的	8A
portal /ˈpɔːt(ə)l/	*n.*	a doorway, gate, or other entrance, especially a large and imposing one 大门, 入口	2A

postoperative /ˌpəʊstˈɒp(ə)rətɪv/	*a.*	during, relating to, or denoting the period following a surgical operation 手术后的	7A
postulate /ˈpɒstjʊleɪt/	*n.*	a thing suggested or assumed as true as the basis for reasoning, discussion, or belief 假定，基本原理	6A
practitioner /prækˈtɪtʃ(ə)nə/	*n.*	执业医生；从业者(尤指律师、医师)	1L
precise /prɪˈsaɪs/	*a.*	marked by exactness and accuracy of expression or detail 明确的；确切的	1B
preclude /prɪˈkluːd/	*vt.*	prevent from happening; make impossible 妨碍；阻止	7A
predispose /ˌpriːdɪˈspəʊz/	*vt.*	make it likely that you will suffer from a particular illness 使易患病	5B
preeminent /priːˈemɪnənt/	*a.*	surpassing all others; very distinguished in some way 杰出的，出色的	7B
premature /ˈpremətʃə/	*a.*	occurring or done before the usual or proper time; too early 过早的，提前的	6A
preparation /ˌprepəˈreɪʃ(ə)n /	*n.*	制剂	7L
prerequisite /priːˈrekwɪzɪt/	*n.*	a prior condition for sth. else to happen or exist 先决条件	2B
prescribe /prɪˈskraɪb/	*vt.*	(of a medical practitioner) advise and authorize the use of (a medicine or treatment) for someone, especially in writing 开处方	2A
prescription /prɪˈskrɪpʃ(ə)n/	*n.*	an instruction written by a medical practitioner that authorizes a patient to be issued with a medicine or treatment 药方，处方	1A
prevail /prɪˈveɪl/	*vi.*	prove more powerful or superior 战胜，占上风	2A
priority /praɪˈɒrɪti/	*n.*	the fact or condition of being regarded or treated as more important than others 优先考虑的事；优先，优先权	1A
privacy /ˈprɪvəsi/	*n.*	a state in which one is not observed or disturbed by other people 隐私，不受公众干扰的状态	8B
privileged /ˈprɪvəlɪdʒd/	*a.*	having special rights or advantages that most people do not have 享有特权的；特许的，专用的	1B
problematic /ˌprɒbləˈmætɪk/	*a.*	constituting or presenting a problem 成问题的，产生问题的	1A
proclaim /prəˈkleɪm/	*vt.*	announce officially or publicly (正式)宣布，(公开)声明	8A
productive /prəˈdʌktɪv/	*a.*	(of a cough) that raises mucus from the respiratory tract 多产的	3A
professionalism /prəˈfeʃ(ə)n(ə)lɪz(ə)m/	*n.*	the competence or skill expected of a professional 职业水准或特性	8B
profuse /prəˈfjuːs/	*a.*	very plentiful, abundant 丰富的，大量的	2B
prognosis /prɒɡˈnəʊsɪs/	*n.*	a forecast of the likely outcome of a situation 预测；[医]预后	5B
prohibitive /prə(ʊ)ˈhɪbɪtɪv/	*a.*	(指价格等)过高的	7L
proliferation /prəˌlɪfəˈreɪʃn/	*n.*	rapid increase in the number or amount of sth. 激增；剧增	6A
prolonged /prəˈlɒŋd/	*a.*	continuing for a long time or longer than usual 延长的	3A

promulgator /ˈprɒm(ə)lgeɪtə/	n.	a person who promotes or makes widely known (an idea or cause) 颁布者，公布者	8A
psychiatric /ˌsaɪkɪˈætrɪk/	a.	relating to mental illness or its treatment 精神疾病的	7B
psychosomatic /ˌsaɪkə(ʊ)səˈmætɪk/	a.	(of a physical illness or other condition) caused or aggravated by a mental factor such as internal conflict or stress 受心理影响的	6A
puberty /ˈpjuːbəti/	n.	the period during which adolescents reach sexual maturity and become capable of reproduction 青春期	5B
pungent /ˈpʌn(d)ʒ(ə)nt/	a.	having a sharply strong taste or smell 辛辣的	2A
purgative /ˈpəːgətɪv/	a.	strongly laxative in effect 通便的，泻下的	1A
	n.	a laxative 泻药(药力强)	
pus /pʌs/	n.	a thick yellowish or greenish liquid that is produced in an infected wound 脓	4A
quackery /ˈkwækəri/	n.	dishonest practices and claims to have special knowledge and skill in some field, typically medicine 庸医的医术	8A
quantifiable /ˌkwɒntɪˈfaɪəb(ə)l/	a.	able to be expressed or measured as a quantity 可量化的	1B
radial /ˈreɪdɪəl/	a.	relating to the radius 桡骨的	3B
radiate /ˈreɪdieɪt/	vi.	(of light, heat, or other energy) be emitted in the form of rays or waves 辐射；发散	4A
rampage /ræmˈpeɪdʒ/	vi.	(especially of a large group of people) move through a place in a violent and uncontrollable manner 狂暴地乱冲	1B
rave /reɪv/	vi.	talk incoherently, as if one were delirious or mad 胡言乱语，咆哮	2B
receptor /rɪˈseptə/	n.	an organ or cell able to respond to light, heat, or other external stimulus and transmit a signal to a sensory nerve 受体	5A
recipe /ˈresɪpi/	n.	a set of instructions for preparing a particular dish, including a list of the ingredients required 食谱	6B
recklessly /ˈreklɪsli/	ad.	without regard to the danger or the consequences of one's actions; rashly 不在乎地，不顾一切地	8A
recruitment /rɪˈkruːtm(ə)nt/	n.	the action of enlisting new people in the armed forces 补充，招聘	7B
reflect /rɪˈflekt/	vt.	表达，显示	3L
regime /reɪˈʒiːm/	n.	a method or system of organizing or managing sth. 方法	5A
registry /ˈredʒɪstri/	n.	a place where registers or records are kept 记录，登记	8B
relic /ˈrelɪk/	n.	an object, a tradition, etc. that has survived from a period of time that no longer exists 遗迹	4A
remission /rɪˈmɪʃ(ə)n/	n.	a temporary diminution of the severity of disease or pain 减轻，缓和	5B
render /ˈrendə/	vt.	represent and depict artistically 表达；描绘	1B
repose /rɪˈpəʊz/	vt.	(literary) lay sth. to rest in or on [书面语] 将……寄托于，安放在……	8A

respiratory tract	*n.*	呼吸道	5L
restore /rɪˈstɔː/	*vt.*	使恢复，修复	3L
retaliate /rɪˈtælɪeɪt/	*vi.*	make an attack in return for a similar attack 报复，反击	8B
retention /rɪˈtenʃ(ə)n/	*n.*	failure to eliminate a substance from the body 滞留	3A
rhinitis /raɪˈnaɪtɪs/	*n.*	a condition in which the inside of the nose becomes swollen and sore, caused by an infection or an allergy 鼻炎	5B
rhythmically /ˈrɪðmɪkli/	*ad.*	in a rhythmic manner 有节奏地	4B
rigorous /ˈrɪg(ə)rəs/	*a.*	extremely thorough and careful 严密的；缜密的；严格的	8A
robust /rə(ʊ)ˈbʌst/	*a.*	strong and healthy; vigorous 健壮的；精力充沛的	1B
ruddy /ˈrʌdi/	*a.*	(of a person's face) having a healthy red color 红润的，血色好的	1B
runny /ˈrʌnɪ/	*a.*	(of a person's nose) producing or discharging mucus; running (鼻)流涕的	5B
scalpel /ˈskælp(ə)l/	*n.*	a knife with a small, sharp blade, as used by a surgeon 外科手术刀	1B
sciatic /saɪˈætɪk/	*a.*	of or affecting the sciatic nerve; suffering from or liable to sciatica 臀部的；坐骨的；坐骨神经的	7A
sciatica /saɪˈætɪkə/	*n.*	pain in the back, hip and outer side of the leg, caused by pressure on the sciatic nerve 坐骨神经痛	4B
scorpion /ˈskɔːpɪən/	*n.*	a small creature like an insect with eight legs, two front claws (curved and pointed arms) and a long tail that curves over its back and can give a poisonous sting 蝎子	5A
scrape /skreɪp/	*vt.*	remove sth. from a surface by moving sth. sharp and hard like a knife across it 刮	4A
scrupulous /ˈskruːpjʊləs/	*a.*	(of a person or process) careful, thorough, and extremely attentive to details 严谨的；小心的	8A
self-contained /ˌself kənˈteɪnd/	*a.*	(of a thing) complete, or having all that is needed, in itself 自我完备的	1B
senility /sɪˈnɪlɪti/	*n.*	behaving in a confused or strange way, and being unable to remember things, because you are old 衰老的状态	6A
sensation /senˈseɪʃn/	*n.*	a feeling that you get when sth. affects your body 感觉；知觉	4A
sensibility /ˌsensɪˈbɪlɪti/	*n.*	the quality of being able to appreciate and respond to complex emotional or aesthetic influence 感悟(力)，感受(力)	1B
sensitivity /ˌsensɪˈtɪvɪti/	*n.*	the ability to understand other people's feelings 敏感；灵敏性	6A
septal /ˈsept(ə)l/	*a.*	relating to a septum (隔膜) or septa 隔膜的，间隔的	7A
sequela /sɪˈkwiːlə/	*n.*	(*pl.* sequelae) a condition which is the consequence of a previous disease or injury 后遗症	4B
serenity /sɪˈrenɪti/	*n.*	the state of being calm, peaceful, and untroubled 宁静，平静	6A

serotonin /ˌserəˈtəʊnɪn/	n.	a compound present in blood platelets and serum, which constricts the blood vessels and acts as a neurotransmitter 血清素	7A
session /ˈseʃ(ə)n/	n.	（一次）治疗	4L
severe /sɪˈvɪə/	a.	(of sth. bad or undesirable) very great 严重的	3A
shaft /ʃɑːft/	n.	a long thin piece of wood or metal that forms part of a spear axe, golf club, or other object 柄；杆	4A
sift /sɪft/	vi.	examine sth. thoroughly so as to isolate that which is most important and useful 筛选，遴选	3B
simplicity /sɪmˈplɪsɪti/	n.	the quality or condition of being easy to understand or do 简单	3B
sinew /ˈsɪnjuː/	n.	a piece of tough fibrous tissue uniting muscle to bone 肌腱	4B
slimy /ˈslaɪmɪ/	a.	covered by or resembling slime 黏滑的	5B
slippery /ˈslɪp(ə)ri/	a.	(of a surface or an object) difficult to hold firmly or stand on because it is smooth, wet, or slimy 滑的	2A
sluggish /ˈslʌgɪʃ/	a.	不活泼的；无精打采的	6L
soothing /ˈsuːðɪŋ/	a.	慰藉的；使人宽心的	6L
sophisticated /səˈfɪstɪkeɪtɪd/	a.	(of a machine, system, or technique) developed to a high degree of complexity（机器、装置等）高级的，精密的；（方法）复杂的	1A
spasm /ˈspæz(ə)m/	n.	a sudden involuntary muscular contraction or convulsive movement 痉挛；抽搐	4B
spontaneous /spɒnˈteɪnɪəs/	a	(of a process or event) occurring without apparent external cause 自发的	2B
sporadic /spəˈrædɪk/	a.	occurring at irregular intervals or only in a few places; scattered or isolated 不定时的；零星的	7A
sprout /spraʊt/	n.	a shoot of a plant 发芽	2B
squeeze /skwiːz/	vt.	firmly press (sth. soft or yielding), typically with one's fingers 挤，榨	6B
stagnation /stægˈneɪʃ(ə)n/	n.	the state of not flowing or moving 淤塞，停滞	2B
stainless /ˈsteɪnləs/	a.	resistant to discoloration, especially discoloration resulting from corrosion 防锈的	4A
stark /stɑːk/	a.	unpleasantly or sharply clear（对比）鲜明的	3B
stasis /ˈsteɪsɪs/	n.	a stoppage of flow of a body fluid 瘀积	2A
state-of-the-art /ˌsteɪt əv ðɪ ˈɑːt/	a.	the most recent stage in the development of a product, incorporating the newest ideas and features 使用最先进技术的；体现最高水平的	1A
stave /steɪv/	vi.	avert or delay sth. bad or dangerous 避免，延缓	6A
stem /stem/	vi.	originate in or be caused by 源于	2A
stenosis /stɪˈnəʊsɪs/	n.	the abnormal narrowing of a passage in the body 狭窄	7A
stiffness /ˈstɪfnəs/	n.	inability to move easily and without pain 僵硬，强直	4B
stimulus /ˈstɪmjʊləs/	n.	a thing or event that evokes a specific functional reaction in an organ or tissue 刺激物	5A

stir-fry /ˈstə: fraɪ/	vt.	fry (meat, fish, or vegetables) rapidly over a high heat while stirring briskly 用旺火煸，用旺火炒	6B
stool /stu:l/	n.	a piece of solid waste from your body 粪便	5B
strategy /ˈstrætɪdʒi/	n.	a plan of action designed to achieve a long-term or overall aim 策略	3A
striation /straɪˈeɪʃ(ə)n/	n.	the state marked with striae 纹理	2A
stroke /strəʊk/	n.	a sudden disabling attack or loss of consciousness caused by an interruption in the flow of blood to the brain, especially through thrombosis 脑卒中	6A
stutter /ˈstʌtə/	n.	a tendency to talk with continued involuntary repetition of sounds 结巴	2B
subordinate /səˈbɔ:dɪnət/	a.	lower in rank or position 下级的，附属的	2B
subside /səbˈsaɪd/	vi.	become less intense, violent, or severe 减弱	3A
subtle /ˈsʌt(ə)l/	a.	(especially of a change or distinction) so delicate or precise as to be difficult to analyze or describe 不易察觉的；不明显的	3B
superficial /ˌsu:pəˈfɪʃ(ə)l/	a.	existing or occurring at or on the surface 表层的	3B
supervision /ˌsu:pəˈvɪʒn/	n.	the work or activity involved in being in charge of sb./sth. and making sure that everything is done correctly, safely, etc. 监督；管理	6A
supplementary /ˌsʌplɪˈmentri/	a.	provided in addition to sth. else in order to improve or complete it 补充的；额外的	4A
supplementation /ˌsʌplɪmenˈteɪʃ(ə)n/	n.	a thing added to sth. else in order to complete or enhance it 增补	2A
surfeit /ˈsə:fɪt/	n.	an excessive amount of sth. 过度	2A
susceptibility /sə,septɪˈbɪlɪti/	n.	the state or act of being likely or liable to be influenced or harmed by a particular thing 易受影响或损害的状态	2B
swap /swɔp/	vt.	take part in an exchange of 交换	4B
sympathetic /ˌsɪmpəˈθetɪk/	a.	交感神经的	5L
synopsis /sɪˈnɔpsɪs/	n.	a brief summary or general survey of sth. 提要，概要	1A
synthesis /ˈsɪnθɪsɪs/	n.	the combination of components or elements to form a connected whole 综合，合成	2A
synthetic /sɪnˈθetɪk/	a.	(of a substance) made by chemical synthesis, especially to imitate a natural product 综合的，合成的	1B
tablet /ˈtæblɪt/	n.	片剂，药片	7L
taint /teɪnt/	vt.	affect with a bad or undesirable quality 使变质；败坏；玷污	8A
tap /tæp/	vt.	hit sb./sth. quickly and lightly 轻敲	4A
tendon /ˈtenden/	n.	a flexible but inelastic（无弹性的）cord of strong fibrous collagen tissue attaching a muscle to a bone 肌腱	4B
terminology /ˌtə:mɪˈnɔlədʒi/	n.	the body of terms used with a particular technical application in a subject of study, theory, profession, etc. 术语	1B

tetralogy /tɪˈtrælədʒi/	n.	a set of four related symptoms or abnormalities frequently occurring together 四联症	7A
texture /ˈtekstʃə/	n.	the feel, appearance, or consistency of a surface or a substance 质地	3B
therapeutic /ˌθerəˈpjuːtɪk/	a.	relating to the healing of disease 治疗(学)的,疗法的	1A
therapy /ˈθerəpi/	n.	治疗	1L
thoracotomy /ˌθɔːrəˈkɔtəmɪ/	n.	surgical incision into the chest wall 开胸手术	4A
throb /θrɔb/	vi.	feel pain in a series of regular beats 抽痛	3B
thrust /θrʌst/	vt.	push a pointed object into sb./sth. with a sudden strong movement 插;戳	4A
thyroidectomy /ˌθaɪrɔiˈdektəmi/	n.	removal of the thyroid gland by surgery 甲状腺切除术	7A
tilt /tɪlt/	vt.	cause to move into a sloping position 使倾斜	4B
tonification /ˌtəʊnɪfɪˈkeɪʃ(ə)n/	n.	(of acupuncture or herbal medicine) the effect or the function of increasing the available energy of (a bodily part or system) 补益,强壮	1A
tonify /ˈtəʊnɪfaɪ/	vt.	(of acupuncture or herbal medicine) increase the available energy of (a bodily part or system) 补养,补益	3A
tonsillectomy /ˌtɔnsɪˈlektəmi/	n.	a surgical operation to remove the tonsils 扁桃体切除术	7A
torso /ˈtɔːsəʊ/	n.	the trunk of the human body 躯干	3B
trance /trɑːns/	n.	a half-conscious state characterized by an absence of response to external stimuli, typically as induced by hypnosis (催眠) or entered by a medium 出神;恍惚	6A
tranquility /trænˈkwɪləti/	n.	the state of being quiet and peaceful 平静,安静	6A
tranquilizer /ˈtræŋkwɪlaɪzə/	n.	a medicinal drug taken to reduce tension or anxiety 镇静剂	7A
transformation /ˌtrænsfəˈmeɪʃ(ə)n/	n.	转化	2L
treatise /ˈtriːtɪs/	n.	a written work dealing formally and systematically with a subject 论述;专著	1A
tremor /ˈtremə/	n.	an involuntary quivering movement 震颤	5A
tuberculosis /tjuˌbəːkjʊˈləʊsɪs/	n.	an infectious bacterial disease characterized by the growth of nodules (tubercles) in the tissues, especially the lungs 肺结核	7A
turbid /ˈtəːbɪd/	a.	cloudy, opaque, or thick with suspended matter 浑浊的	2A
turmeric /ˈtəːmərɪk/	n.	a bright yellow aromatic powder obtained from the rhizome of a plant of the ginger family, used for flavoring and coloring in Asian cooking and formerly as a fabric dye 姜黄	6B
twirl /twɜːl/	vt.	spin quickly and lightly round, especially repeatedly 捻转	4A
ulcer /ˈʌlsə/	n.	a sore area on the outside of the body or on the surface of an organ inside the body which is painful and may bleed or produce a poisonous substance 溃疡	1B
ulna /ˈʌlnə/	n.	(pl. ulnae; ulnas) the thinner and longer of the two bones in the human forearm, on the side opposite to the thumb 尺骨	4B

ultimate /ˈʌltɪmət/	*a.*	being or happening at the end of a process; final 最后的	3A
unauthorized /ʌnˈɔːθəraɪzd/	*a.*	not having official permission or approval 未经授权的；未经许可的	8B
unlicensed /ʌnˈlaɪs(ə)nst/	*a.*	无执照的，无资格证的	7L
unobstructed /ˌʌnəbˈstrʌktɪd/	*a.*	不被阻塞的，畅通无阻的	1L
upbearing /ʌpˈbeərɪŋ/	*n.*	turning and proceeding in an upward direction 向上	2A
uphold /ʌpˈhəuld/	*vt.*	confirm or support (sth. which has been questioned) 支持；赞成；支撑	8B
urethra /juˈriːθrə/	*n.*	the duct by which urine is conveyed out of the body from the bladder, and which in male vertebrates also conveys semen 尿道	2A
urgency /ˈəːdʒ(ə)nsi/	*n.*	importance requiring swift action 紧急	3A
urine /ˈjuərɪn/	*n.*	a watery, typically yellowish fluid stored in the bladder and discharged through the urethra 尿	1B
uterus /ˈjuːt(ə)rəs/	*n.*	(*pl.* uteri or uteruses) the organ in the lower body of a woman or female mammal where offspring are conceived and in which they gestate (孕育) before birth 子宫	3A
vegetarian /ˌvedʒɪˈteərɪən/	*n.*	a person who does not eat meat or fish, and sometimes other animal products, especially for moral, religious, or health reasons 素食者	6B
veil /veɪl/	*n.*	a piece of fine material worn by women to protect or conceal the face 面纱	3B
vein /veɪn/	*n.*	静脉，脉	2L
velocity /vɪˈlɔsɪti/	*n.*	the speed of sth. in a given direction 速率，速度	5A
ventricular /ˈventrɪkjulə/	*a.*	of or relating to a ventricle (室) of the heart 心室的	7A
vexation /vekˈseɪʃ(ə)n/	*n.*	the state of being annoyed, frustrated, or worried 心烦，忧虑，恼怒	2B
vibrate /vaɪˈbreɪt/	*vt.*	make sth. move from side to side very quickly and with small movements 使振动；使颤动	4A
viral /ˈvaɪr(ə)l/	*a.*	病毒的	5L
virtuous /ˈvəːtʃuəs/	*a.*	品德高的；善良的	8L
vitalize /ˈvaɪt(ə)laɪz/	*vt.*	give strength and energy to 激发	5A
warrant /ˈwɔr(ə)nt/	*vt.*	justify or necessitate (a course of action) 保证	3A
weed /wiːd/	*vt.*	remove an inferior or unwanted component of a group or collection 消除	8A
whoop /wuːp/	*vi.*	make the paroxysmal (阵发性) gasp characteristic of whooping cough 喘息	3A
yardstick /ˈjɑːdstɪk/	*n.*	a standard used for comparison 码尺；尺度	8B

Note: 1L means the word can be found in the Listening part of Unit 1, and 2L in that of U2; 1A means Text A of Unit 1; 2A means Text A of Unit 2; 1B means Text B of Unit 1; 2B means Text B of Unit 2; so on and so forth.

Appendix IV

Phrases and Expressions

Phrases and Expressions	Chinese Meaning	Unit
a cause of further pathology	继发性病理因素	3A
a follow-up study	追踪研究	5A
a socially embarrassing disease	尴尬难言的疾病	8B
a system of great depth	深奥的体系	8A
abdominal pain	腹痛	4A
abide by the ethical code of the TCM profession	遵守中医行业的道德准则	8B
account for	对……负有责任;导致;(比例)占	2A
accumulation of phlegm	痰积	5B
acquit oneself of	宣告某人无罪;原谅某人	8A
acupuncture anesthesia	针刺麻醉	4A
acupuncture anesthesia/analgesia	针刺麻醉 / 镇痛	7A
acute attack	急性发作	5B
acute episode	急性发作	5B
acute illness	急性病	6A
adhere to the laws	遵循法律	8B
advanced tuberculosis	肺结核晚期	7A
advisory body	咨询机构	4L
aerobic conditioning	有氧运动	6A
affiliated hospital	附属医院	1A
agents of disease	病原体	1B
allergic disorder	过敏性疾病	7B
alleviate pain	缓解疼痛	4A
anus and the urethra	二阴	2A
approved continuing education	经过认证的继续教育	8A
arouse interest	引发……兴趣	7A
as a consequence	因此	7B
as per usual practice	照例	5A
asthmatic episode	哮喘发作	5L
at a moderate pace	以适度的速度	4B

at large	整体上,总体上	8B
at one's own discretion	依据,随某人的意愿处理	8A
balance of yin and yang	阴阳平衡,阴平阳秘	6A
be adept at	擅长,善于	6A
be ascribed to	归结于	2A
be classified into	分类为	3B
be consistent with	与……一致的,和谐的	8A
be dedicated to + v-ing/sth.	致力于……	8B
be diverted from	使分心	8A
be essential for	对……来说重要	6B
be given in two doses per day	每日两剂	5A
be in excess	过盛	2B
be incorporated into	合并到……,被整合到……	8A
be inherently supportive of	从本质(根本)上支持	8A
be liable to	易于……	8A
be rooted in	根植于……,源于……	1B
be secondary to	是次要的	1B
be unique to	属于特定(人或者地方)的,具有特定风格的	8A
birth history	生育史	3B
blood flow velocity	血流速度	5A
blood stagnation	血滞	2B
blood sugar level	血糖水平	6A
body fluid	津液	2B
bowel movement	排便	3B
breech fetal position	胎儿臀位	7A
broncho-dilating medication	支气管扩张药	5B
but not limited to	但不限于……	1A
cause and effect	因果(关系)	1B
center around	以……为中心	3B
characterize... as...	把……的特征描述为……	1B
Chinese herbal medicine	中草药,中药	1A
chop up	切细,切断	6B
chronic bronchitis	慢性支气管炎	7A
chronic condition	慢性病	6A
chronic obstructive pulmonary disease	慢性阻塞性肺疾病	7A
chronic pain management	慢性疼痛控制	7B
clear yang	清阳	2A
clearing lung-heat and resolving phlegm	清肺化痰	3A
clinical practice	临床实践	1A
clinical presentation	临床表现	5B
coexistence of deficiency and excess	虚实夹杂	3A
coincide with	同时发生	3A

cold congealing in the uterus	寒凝胞宫	3A
cold-damp obstruction	寒湿痹阻	4A
come alive	活跃起来	6B
continuing education	继续教育	7A
conventional medication	常规药物	7A
convert into	转变为,转化为	1A
cool down	冷却;平静下来	6B
copious perspiration	多汗	2B
copious white watery phlegm	大量的白稀痰	5B
cotton gauze	纱布辅料	4A
critical thinking	批判性思维	1B
cultural affiliation	文化归属	1B
curative potential	治愈潜能	6A
damp heat affecting the spleen	湿热困脾	1B
deal with ethical conflicts	处理伦理冲突	8B
decreased appetite	食欲下降	5B
deep-lying phlegm	伏痰	5B
deficiency of both qi and blood	气血两虚	3A
deficient yin affecting the stomach	胃阴虚(证)	1B
dental operation	牙科手术	7A
derive from	源于;衍生于	2A
develop its own perception of health and illness	对健康与疾病形成独特的认识	1B
diagnosis and treatment	诊断与治疗	1A
diagnosis of the face	面诊	3B
diagnostic technique	诊断技术	1B
dietary therapy	饮食疗法	1A
differentiation of patterns	辨证	1A
dispel the evil and support the good	祛邪扶正	1L
dominant hand	惯用手,优势手	4A
dopaminergic receptor stimulant	多巴胺受体兴奋剂	5A
dredge meridians	疏通经络	4A
dry cough	干咳	3A
during the period	月经期间	3A
dynamic equilibrium	动态平衡	6A
ebb away	渐渐衰退;消逝	6B
elective course	选修课	7A
eliminate edema	消肿	3A
endocrine disorder	内分泌紊乱	1B
enjoy the trust of the society	得到社会的信任	8B
environmental exposure	环境暴露(接触)	5B
epigastric pain	胃脘痛	4A
essence of grain and water	水谷精微	2B

ethical code	道德准则	8B
ethical committee	伦理委员会	8B
even with best of intentions	即使出于最好的目的	8A
excess fire	实火	1B
extensive clinical observation and testing	大量的临床观察和检验	1B
extensor muscle	伸肌	4B
exterior invasion of a pathogenic factor	外感病邪	3A
fade from	消退;减退	7A
far beyond the basics learned in a college program	远远超出大学课程中学到的基础知识	8A
feel the pulse	把脉	2A
filiform needle	毫针	4A
five phases	五行	1A
five *zang*-organs	五脏	2A
food therapy	食疗	6B
for personal gain	为了(谋取)个人利益	8B
four examinations (of diagnosis)	四诊	3B
four methods of diagnosis	四诊	3L
frequent urination	尿频	5A
from sb.'s perspective	从……的角度看	1B
frozen shoulder	五十肩,肩凝症	4B
gain (more) understanding of sth.	对……有(更多的)理解,增进理解	1A
gain popularity	得到普及	1A
gall bladder	胆囊	3B
general principle	基本原则	6B
get a depth of knowledge	深入了解(获得)知识	8A
get right	清楚无误地了解	4B
get to grips with	对付;掌握要领	4B
give priority to	认为……优先,优先考虑	1A
give rise to	引起	2B
govern blood and vessels	主血脉	2B
have no basis in	在某方面没有(理论)基础	8A
have trust and confidence in the TCM profession	对中医专业建立信任和信心	8B
health care	保健	1A
heart blood depletion	心血耗竭	2B
herbal formula	方剂	3B
high dose	大剂量	7A
higher incidences of allergic rhinitis	过敏性鼻炎发生率较高	5B
holistic approach concept	整体观	1A
imbalance and blockage	失衡和阻滞	6A
in a professional manner	以专业的方式	8B
in accordance with the standards	符合标准	8A
in confidence	私下	8B

in conjunction with	与……协力	5B
in contrast	与此相反；相比之下	1B
in its own way	按其自身的方式	6B
in line with	与……一致，符合	1A
in place	在恰当的位置	4B
in professionally supervised clinics	在有专业人员指导的诊所	8A
in the country of origin	在起（发）源国家	8A
in the course of their practice	在行医过程中	8B
index finger	食指	4A
induct and deduct	归纳和演绎	1A
infectious disease	传染病	6A
inflammatory process	炎性过程	5A
initial form	雏形，最初形式	4A
inspect the complexion	望面色	2A
internal vigor	机体活力	6A
internal wind	内风	5A
interrupted pulse	结代脉	2B
keep abreast of	跟上	8B
keep confidential all medical information	保守医疗信息秘密	8B
keep firmly the ethical code in mind	将道德准则牢记在心	8B
key reference material	主要参考资料	7B
lassitude of spirit	神疲	2B
laws and regulations governing TCM practice	中医医疗行业的法规和条例	8B
like hell	拼命地	3B
looking diagnosis	望诊	3B
lumbosacral region	腰骶部	4A
lusterless complexion	色悴	5B
main complaint	主诉	3B
map... onto	映射到	3B
massive pulmonary embolism	大面积肺栓塞	7A
medical emergency	急诊	6A
medical modality	治疗方式；医学模式	7A
medicinal cuisine	药膳	6B
medicinal effect	药用效果	6B
menstrual cycle	月经周期	3B
mental faculty	智力，智能	2B
metabolic rate	代谢率	6A
miniature adult	成人的微缩版	5B
move blood and stop pain	行血止痛	3A
needle retention	留针	5A
needling sensation	得气	4A
Neolithic archaeological site	新石器时代考古遗址	4A

neurological disorder	神经系统疾病,神经障碍,神经紊乱	1B
neuron degeneration	神经元变性	5A
night sweating	盗汗	2B
nourish blood	养血	2A
on humanitarian basis	基于人道主义精神	8B
on staff	在职;在岗	7A
on the go	活跃,忙个不停	1B
out of balance	失衡,失调	6B
oversee criteria	监督标准	7B
pain management	疼痛治疗	7A
palpation of the abdomen	按腹	3B
palpation of the acupuncture meridians	按经络	3B
pathogenic and healthy qi	邪气和正气	2A
pathogenic factor	邪气;致病因素	1A
pattern of disharmony	病证	1B
pediatric asthma	小儿哮喘	5B
phlegm obstruction	痰阻	5A
physical strength	体力	6A
physiological and psychological	生理与心理的	1B
pivotal point	轴心,中心点	4B
posterior aspect	后侧	4B
precise cause	确切病因	1B
prevent liver wind from going to the head	防止肝风上扰	1B
preventative measure	预防措施	6A
pride... on	对……感到自豪	5B
provide the framework for treatment	提供治疗框架	1B
pulmonary edema	肺水肿	7A
pulmonary fibrosis	肺纤维化	7A
qi not holding blood	气不摄血	3A
qi stagnation	气滞	4B
quality assurance	质量保障	7B
quality of the pain	疼痛性质	3B
radial artery	桡动脉	3B
refer to	指的是……;提到	8A
remission stage	缓解期	5B
remove pus	排脓	4A
reside in	居住,存在于	6A
respiratory tract	呼吸道	5L
retention of phlegm in the lung	痰浊阻肺	3A
scarring moxibustion	瘢痕灸	4A
second best to	仅次于	8L
separate entity	独立体	3A

shortness of breath	气短	2B
six *fu*-organs	六腑	2A
slippery pulse	脉滑	3A
slippery rapid pulse	脉象滑数	5B
speak highly of sth.	高度赞扬	4A
specialize in	专门研究	3B
spleen deficiency and dampness	脾虚夹湿	3A
spontaneous sweating	自汗	2B
sprout of the heart	心之苗	2B
stainless steel	不锈钢	4A
stasis of blood	血瘀	3A
statutory regulation	法令规范,法令规则	7B
stave off	延缓;推迟	6A
stem from	起源于	2A
stop the cough	止咳	3A
store the spirit	藏神	2B
stress-related disorder	压力性疾病,应激性疾病	7B
stroke rehabilitation	脑卒中康复	7A
supply of blood	供血	2B
susceptibility to fright	易惊	2B
symptoms and signs	症状与体征	1B
take precautions against	对……采取预防措施	8A
tender areas	压痛点	3L
tennis elbow	网球肘	4B
the doctrine of the golden mean	中庸之道	1A
the right to be informed	知情权	8B
the right to privacy and dignity	隐私权和尊严	8B
the scope of TCM practice	中医行医范围	8A
the therapeutic regime for Parkinson's disease	帕金森病的治疗方案	5A
theoretical framework	理论框架	1A
therapeutic effect	疗效	7A
therapeutic method	治法	1A
thought and practice	思想与实践	1B
tightness in the chest	胸闷	5B
to name a few	举几个例子	1A
tolerance limit	耐受限度	5A
tongue coating	舌苔	3A
tonic spasm	强直性痉挛	5A
trace back to	追溯到	7B
track and field	田径	7A
turbid yin	浊阴	2A
turtle-shell artifact	龟甲制品	6A

251

twelve (of the main) meridians	十二正经	3B
two aspects of a contradiction	矛盾的两个方面	3A
under the heading of	以……为标题	8A
underlying mechanism	潜在机制	1B
upper portals	上窍	2A
vital energy	生命力,气	6A
vital essence	精华	6A
ward off	预防	6A
warm and supplement yang qi	温补阳气	2A
watch out	当心	4B
wax and wane	起伏,起落,消长	7A
whooping cough	百日咳	3A
within the accredited courses	在认可(学分)的课程之内	8A
without prejudice of race	没有种族偏见	8B
without proof	没有依据,没有证据	8A
without the patient's consent	未经患者同意	8B
yin and yang pathogens	阴邪和阳邪	2A
yin-yang imbalance	阴阳失调	2A
zero in on	(使)对准……;全神贯注于(问题或主题)	1B

Note: 1A means Text A of Unit 1; 2A means Text A of Unit 2; 1B means Text B of Unit 1; 2B means Text B of Unit 2; so on and so forth.

Appendix V

Word Roots and Affixes

Roots/Affixes	Meaning of Roots/Affixes	Unit
a-	no or without	2B
ab-	go bad	3A
abdomin(o)	abdomen	2A
ac-	more, again	7B
acid	sour	7A
acu-	needle	2A
-ade	forming a noun	6B
adip(o)-	fat	7B
-al	pertaining to	5A
-algia	pain	7A
ana-	apart	2A
anethes(o)	insensitivity	4A
angi(o)	of blood vessel	4B
anti-	against	1B
append(o)	appendix	7A
arch-	ancient	4A
art-/arti-	skill	6A
arteri(o)	of the artery	4B
arthr(o)-	joint	1A
-ary	pertaining to	8B
-ase	enzyme	8A
-asthenia	weakness	2A
athero	of or pertaining to arteriosclerosis	5A
atri(o)	atrium	7A
-atric	treat, medical healing	5A
bi(o)	life	1A
bi-/di-	two,double	8B
brach(i)	arm	6B
brady-	slow	8A
bronch(o)	windpipe	5B
-bustion	burning	4A

calc(o)/calci(o)	calcium	8A
carb	carbon	4A
cardi(o)	heart	3B
cauli	caudex	6B
cept	take	5A
cerebr(o)	of the brain	4B
chem(o)	chemistry	7A
chol	gallbladder	5A
chron(o)	time	3B
cide	kill	2A
circ	circle	3B
circum-	around	1B
cise	cut	6B
clast	to break, destroy	8A
co-	together	3A
col	with, together	7B
contra-	opposite	3A
coron	crown	6B
cortic(o)	of the adrenal or cerebral cortices	4B
counter-	against; opposite	2A
crani(o)	relating to the cranium	4B
crin(o)	secretion, the production of a substance	1B
cruit	grow	7B
cry(o)	cold	2A
cuis/cuit	cook	6B
-cular	pertaining to	4A
curr-	run	7B
cyst(o)	of the urinary bladder	4B
cyt(o)/cyte	cell	8A
de-	reduce	3A
dem(o)	connected with people or population	1A
dent(o)	teeth	8A
dext	the right-hand side	4A
dia-	through	3A
dict	say, assert	
dif-	separate	3B
dis-	lack of; not	1B
doc-	teach	1A
dual	double	2A
-dynia	pain	3B
dys-	bad	3A
-ectomy	removal	4A
electro	electricity	4A
-emia	blood condition	3B

en-	put into or on	1A
-en	cause to be	5B
-ence	action, process	5A
endo-	within	1B
enter(o)	small intestine	8A
equ	equal, same	6A
erythr(o)-	red, red cell	7B
esthes/esthesi(o)	sense	8A
exo-	outside, outer	1A
exter-	outside	5B
fact	do/make	7B
fasci(o)	fibrous band	7A
femor(o)	relating to the thigh bone	4B
fibr(o)	fiber	6A
fil(i)	thread	4A
flu(o)	flow	3B
fore-	before, in front	3B
forti	strong	5B
fus	pour	2A
gastr(o)	stomach	1B
gen-	line of descent	5A
-gen	that which produces	6B
-genic	causing	2A
gloss(o)	tongue	8A
gluco	relating to glucose	6B
-gnosis	knowledge	5B
-gram	record	3B
granul(o)	granule	7B
-graph	record	1A
grav	heavy	5B
gyn(a)ec(o)-	woman	1A
hal	breath, breathe	5B
hemo/haemato	relating to blood	6B
hepa/hepat	liver	2A
hetero-	different	6B
hex-	six	8B
hidr(o)	perspiration, sweating	4B
holo-	entire, complete	3B
hyper-	excessive	3A
homo-	same	5A
hypno	relating to sleep	6B
hypo-	below, under	3B
hyster(o)	uterus	3A
-ia	disease; pathological or abnormal condition	1B

255

-ic	of	5B
-ics	denoting arts or sciences, branches of study or action	1A
im-	no, not	5B
immun(o)	immunity	6A
in-	not; the opposite or lack of sth.	1B
infra-	under, beneath, below	7A
inter-	inward	3A
-ion	condition, state	7B
ischi(o)	of ischium or hucklebone	4B
iso-	equal	6A
-istic	of or pertaining to	2B
-itude	quality or state	5A
-ity	condition or quality of being...	5B
-ive	related to	7B
ject	throw	6A
junct	join	5B
kine	movement	5A
kyph(o)	hump	7A
labi(o)	lip	3A
labor	labor	7B
-lalia	indicating a speech defect or abnormality	8A
laryng(o)	throat	7B
-less	without	2B
leuk(o)	white	8B
- (o)logy	denoting a subject of study or interest	1A
lithic	stone	4A
-lysis	breakdown, destruction	5A
macro-	large	3B
mal-	in a faulty or inadequate manner	6B
malacia	abnormal softening	8B
mani-/manu	hand	4A
mast(o)	mammary	4B
matur	ripe	5A
mega-	large	6A
men(o)	menstruation	3A
-ment	the act or state or fact of...	5B
meta-	altered	1A
-meter	instrument for, measuring	2A
metro-	mother	6A
micro-	small	3B
mid-	middle	3A
migr-	remove	7B
migra	wander	3B
mill(i)-	thousand	1A

mini-	minor	5B
-mne	memory	5A
mono-	one	1A
multi-	many	3A
muscul(o)	muscle	7A
my(o)	muscle	2B
myel(o)	relating to the marrow of brain and bone	4B
neo-	new	2A
-ness	forming nouns, the state or quality of	3A
neur(o)	nerve	5A
non-	not	2B
nulli	none	6B
odont	teeth	8A
oesophag(o)	esophageal	4B
-oid	-like, like that of	8A
ophthalm(o)	eye	7B
-opsy	view of	2B
or(o)	mouth	8A
orth(o)-	straight, upright	6A
oste(o)	bone	1A
ot(o)	ear	1A
-ous	characterized by; of the nature of	1A
out-	beyond, more than	5B
over-	much	7A
pan-	all, wide	2A
path(o)	disease, illness, sickness	1A
-pathy	disease	3A
ped	child	5B
pend	hang	4A
-penia	decreasing, lack of	8B
pent-	five	8B
-pepsia/-peps	digestion	8A
per-	through	1B
pha/phe	say, speak	2B
phage/phago	eat, swallow	8B
-phasia	speech	8A
phobia	an extreme or irrational fear of or aversion to sth.	4B
physi(o)-	relating to natural forces or function	1B
pict	paint	3B
plasia	development or formation	8B
plasm	the constituent substance of cells	8B
plegia	paralysis; losing feeling in or control of	8B
pleur(o)	of pleura	7A
pneum(o)	air, lung, breathing	1B

pod(o)	foot	7B
poly-	many	6A
potent	power, ability	6A
pre-	before	2B
press	press	1B
pro-	many	2B
pseud(o)-	not genuine; sham	4B
psych(o)	mind	6A
-ptosis	drooping	8B
pub(o)	genital region	7B
pulmon(o)-	lung	7A
puncture	prick	4A
quadri-	four	8B
radi(o)	radius	3B
radi(o)	radiating	4A
re-	again	2B
rect(o)	of the rectum	4B
ren(o)	kidney	2B
rhin(o)	nose	5B
-rrhea	flow, flowing	5A
scend	climb	3A
sciat(o)	sciatic nerve	7A
sclerosis	a hardening of tissue and other anatomical features	4B
-scope	instrument	1B
-scopy	examination	2B
semi-	half, part	3B
sens-	feel	1B
sept-	seven	8B
simil	alike/same	2B
sinus(o)	sinus, cavity	6B
sol	alone	1B
solu/solv	loosen	3A
-some	body	2B
somn(i)	sleep	1B
soph	wise	1A
sphygm(o)	pulse	6A
splen(o)	spleen	8A
sta-	stay, stand still	5A
steth(o)	chest	6A
stomat(o)	mouth	8A
string	tighten	2A
sub-	under	2B
super-	above, over	5B
supra-	upper	2A

syn	join	2A
tachy-	fast	8A
tens	stretch	1B
-tension	pressure	6B
termin	limit	1B
tetra	four	7A
therm(o)	heat, temperature	2A
thorac(o)	thorax	4A
thromb(o)	blood clot	8B
thyr(o)	pertaining to thyroid	7A
tonsill(o)	of the tonsil	4B
top(o)	part	8B
trans-	transfer	3B
tri-	three	8B
troph(o)	nutrition	8B
ultra-	super	2B
- (i)um	denoting singular, grammatical number	5B
-uncle	little, small	4A
under-	below, secondary to	7B
uni-	one	6B
ur(o)	urine	2B
urgy	technology	4A
uter	uterus	3A
valv(o)	valve	6B
vas(o)	vessel	2B
vascul(o)	blood vessel	6A
vege	plant	6B
veloc(i)	speed, swift, rapid	5A
ven(o)	vein	6A
ventricul(o)	ventricle	7A
vibr	swing	4A
vita	life, living	5A
vok	call, voice	7B

Note: 1A means Text A of Unit 1; 2A means Text A of Unit 2; 1B means Text B of Unit 1; 2B means Text B of Unit 2; so on and so forth.

Appendix VI

Listening Scripts, Text Translations and Keys to the Exercises

Unit 1

Unit 2

Unit 3

Unit 4

Unit 5

Unit 6

Unit 7

Unit 8